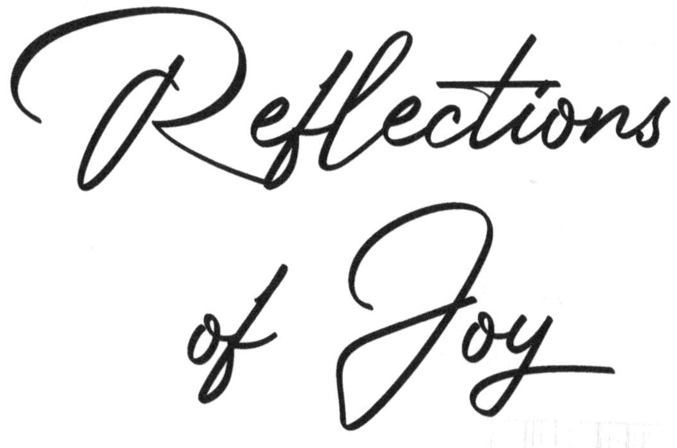

LEARNING TO LOVE THE WOMAN
YOU SEE WHILE BECOMING THE
ONE YOU'RE MEANT TO BE

By

Kim Mosiman

Published by hope*books
2217 Matthews Township Pkwy
Suite D302
Matthews, NC 28105
www.hopebooks.com

hope*books is a division of hope*media

Printed in the United States of America

First paperback edition.
Paperback ISBN: 979-8-89185-030-9
Hardcover ISBN: 979-8-89185-031-6
Ebook ISBN: 979-8-89185-032-3
Library of Congress Number: 2023950993

Bible References use The NIV Study Bible,
Zondervan 1995 except where noted.

To Mom

You are my first memory of love and everything I aspire to be.

I love you.

&

To women everywhere
May you always see your beauty, explore your gifts,
and know you are loved.

Table of Contents

Introduction 3

- Learning to Listen 9
- Crowding Out 10
- The Journey 11

Chapter 1: Give it Up 15

- Faith Journey 15
- Be Careful 24
- Childlike Faith 28
- Take Delight 31
- Do Nothing 37
- Spirit Lead 39
- Crowding Out for Prayer 42

Chapter 2: Write it Down 47

- Owner's Manual 47
- Why Write? 49
- Choose Your Audience 52
- Morning Pages 55
- Write Now 57
- Do It "Write" 59
- Crowding Out to Write 63

Chapter 3: Reflections 65

- Who Are You? 65
- Look In the Mirror 68
- Skip the Scale 71
- The Friend 76
- This is Me 79
- Wonderfully Made 81
- Crowding Out to Simplify Your Look 88

Chapter 4: Up & Down 91

- Breaking Point 91
- Ground Zero 94
- No Pain, No Gain 97
- Love Yourself 100
- Masterpiece 103
- Use it or Lose It 106
- Crowding Out for Movement 110

Chapter 5: Savor 113

- I Can't Eat That! 113
- In Touch 116
- Convenience 119
- Discipline Fatigue 124
- What's On Your Plate? 127
- "Planning Vs. Prepping" 133
- Crowding Out in the Kitchen 138

Chapter 6: Your Calling 143

- Refocus 143

- Nudges 146
- Dream 148
- Simple Gatherings 151
- Family First 154
- Inspiration 158
- Crowding Out For Fellowship 161

Chapter 7: Let Go 165

- For Fun 165
- Gifts 168
- Head Nowhere 170
- Take the Time 173
- Make the Change 175
- Relax 178
- Just Right 181
- Crowding Out for Yourself 183

Conclusion: You Decide 185

- It Can Be Easy 185
- You Can Make it Hard 186
- My Prayer for You 189

The Back of the Book 191

- Kim's 55th Blessing List 191
- Example of Written Journal 192
- Example of Bullet Journal 197
- My Favorite Foods 198
- My Well-Stocked Kitchen 199
- Balanced Examples 200

- Cook Once- Eat Again 201
- Planned Leftovers 203
- Seasonings 208
- Breakfast 209
- Snacks & Appetizers 213
- Soups 217
- Main Dishes 221
- Beverages 224
- Desserts 226

Acknowledgments 229

Citations 231

A note from Kim:

I wish you could see the apple tree that lives so beautifully in my front yard. I'm sure if I could hear her speak, she'd be gasping a long sigh of relief. Her branches were bent almost to the ground with the weight of her fruit, but she held on without a single broken branch, long enough for the apples to reach their sweet-tart, crunchy ripeness.

I'm not a fan of sprays; some apples have bug bumps, wormholes, and a dusty, dingy cast on the peel. Many people would be so bold as to call them rotten and throw them away. Heaven forbid they might take a bite of the delicious fruit, warm from the sun.

I know underneath that battered skin lies perfection. I cut into the unpleasant outside and find beautiful crisp white flesh that can be eaten out of hand, roasted, cooked into sauce, or frozen to be used another day.

It's kind of a talent I have— finding beauty in things that others would throw away. It happened almost every day for more than seven years when I owned a small boutique gym lovingly named My Gym. People walked in the door feeling sad, unhealthy, and, well, ugly. Many had lost the ability to feel 'good enough,' and that's where I came in.

My goal was always to get members to look beyond the mirror (and the scale) because when they do– magical things happen. Learning to celebrate small victories like the reduction of meds and better sleep can be the inspiration we need long before the big goals of weight loss and toned muscles are met. When we look past the surface, there are many ways to find joy in the journey to good health.

There is no perfect in this life– my world is full of dirty clothes, messy counters, stacks of bills, and an overfull calendar. It also includes love and good friends, sunrises, and ugly apples, all of which have the potential to become something sweet and delicious and perfect for me.

In the pages that follow, I'll share my story. There were years when I spiraled out of control in unhealthy ways and felt spiritually lost. Fortunately, I discovered there is a way to get off that path. I pray you'll learn to find the good in yourself, no matter where you're starting from… find joy in your journey, and you'll discover a life that can be better than you've ever imagined.

Be Happy

xoxo

Introduction

The dream of writing a book whispered to me many years ago. I had been peer coaching and leading fitness classes for a while and felt I'd finally found my calling. I searched for a gym that felt like home and trained with the owners to duplicate that experience in a space of my own. I opened a "challenge gym," where new members were pulled in with the lure of big results and the opportunity of a prize at the end of the session. The competition atmosphere was tempered with the promise of lifestyle change and accountability coaching.

I followed in the footsteps of my franchisors and worked tirelessly every day to "be more." I wanted my members to feel like family. I spent countless days hand-holding, counseling, number crunching, and cheering. I changed class schedules to accommodate potential new members and veered from the original programming just to keep people engaged.

Owning the gym seemed like the perfect job. I could pick my hours, do something I loved, and make a difference in the lives of those who joined my program.

I was able to provide a safe space for challengers as they battled chronic disease, obesity, infertility, and low self-esteem. I led members through high-intensity kickboxing workouts, pushing them past the point they could reach themselves. I watched carefully during resistance classes and learned to recognize small changes long before they did as they worked head-down in the plank position or head-up in the overhead press. I trained members who completed the program to do the same, and over time, my gym and our coaching style turned into something special.

The problem arose when this people-pleasing, change-noticing, ever-complementing person let her passion become her purpose. Over several years, my purpose became my job, and, like many of you, I just wanted to go home at the end of the day. Busy days without a workout or a single home-cooked meal turned into weeks, which turned into months. My weight climbed, and my attitude soured.

I opened in February of 2010 and, with the help of many peer coaches, impacted the lives of thousands. It may not sound like a lot, but in the coaching sense, we probably served too many people. In the business sense, it wasn't enough.

I closed the doors in 2017, vowing to stay active and "in touch." I told everyone I was excited to retire and tried to convince myself I was doing the right thing. I thought I would travel more with Jeff and finish projects around home.

The month that followed was spent cleaning out the space. Equipment sales brought former members in to visit, allowing a break in the days I spent sorting through paperwork and memories. Each person who stopped by had already made an imprint on my heart. I remembered their stories and successes, even if I occasionally forgot a name!

After the gym was cleared and I turned the key in the lock for the final time, I spent lazy days sleeping until six! Can you imagine? After almost a decade of 3:50 am alarms, I'd wake up refreshed, wander to the kitchen to make coffee, and snuggle into my favorite chair to read. I read 63 books in the first month! At the time, it seemed indulgent and wonderful. Looking back, this ever-observant coach should have been concerned.

Long, lazy mornings of retirement were just the beginning. I didn't do the things I promised myself. I didn't exercise, cook, or meet my friends for lunch. I didn't visit my parents for coffee or plan a girl's trip with those who vowed to stay in touch. I dove deep down a rabbit hole of wine, food, and lazy days that turned into weeks, months, and years.

My belly was getting squishy, and my legs began to feel fatigued when I climbed the stairs. I was frequently out of breath as a result of treating myself far too often and moving too little.

I spent countless hours planning my return to health, plotting workouts, and recording my food. When the old ways didn't work,

I may have let my "failure" convince me to commit to ridiculous resolutions and torturous methods.

It takes time to create a habit. Maybe I should clarify… It takes time to create a GOOD habit. The bad ones just seem to stop by and stick like glue, don't they? Like many others, I made it a habit to commit to starting over at the turn of a new year or on a birthday. I made promises to myself with my back up against an imaginary wall of mother-of-the-groom dress shopping. I tried to detox my way out of a potential conversation with my doctor, where I knew she would vaguely mention my weight as she tried to stay optimistic about my yearly test results.

Sometime last year, it dawned on me that I had never talked to a client the way I was talking to myself. I didn't encourage them to fast or drink terrible shakes. I didn't tell them to skip out on birthday parties or to give up whole food groups. I didn't assign them tortuous tasks to burn off holiday calories. I helped many people with sound advice, so why couldn't I help myself?

I'm happy to report that I finally saw the light at the end of the tunnel. As it turned out, the light was just the overhead lamp above a cold examination table during my yearly physical. Fortunately, my doctor didn't have to say anything. I told her I was disappointed in my decline and that I'd do what needed to be done.

As I drove home from her office, I thought about all that had changed in the last ten years. The boys were grown and living lives of their own. My gym had closed, and my husband had also sold his business. I rarely had to be anywhere or do anything. I had spiraled out of control, gaining weight and ignoring the signs that my health had taken a turn for the worse. I had become the woman I tried to help all those years at the gym.

I decided to clean things up a bit and treat myself more kindly than I had in the past. I reminded myself it's easier to be healthy when you're happy. It's easier to stick with a program when it's fun. It's easier to eat real food when it's delicious.

I'm attempting to instill habits that include love and respect. My results are a little slower, but I'm sure that they will be forever this time. I look in the mirror and see that my tummy is flatter, and I have one less chin. My skin glows a little more, and I feel myself smiling again.

Wouldn't it be nice if we could all look in the mirror and see past the tired eyes, droopy skin, messy hair, and fat rolls? What if we could see our progress on the inside- stronger muscles, a healthy heart, a well-rested brain? How wonderful would it be to look in the mirror and see all of the good instead of what we've been trained to see?

♥

"Don't be afraid of your fears. They're not there to scare you. They're there to let you know that something is worth it."

— C. JoyBell C.[1]

Every once in a while, I become afraid. Sometimes, it's startling, a silly moment that catches me off guard, or a dream that leaves me unsettled in the dark of the night. Usually, these fears dissipate with the morning light and the busyness that fills my day.

Sometimes, my fear doesn't seem so childlike and doesn't want to go away. It's fierce and protective, and it wants to scream. As I've grown older, I've realized my fear can be tempered by faith. I've learned how important it is to believe in something or someone greater than myself (especially when the world seems to be crumbling around me). Millions of people have lost faith in others, believing only in themselves and relying only on what they can learn or do on their own. My heart tells me we are racing towards a moment when we must believe in others- we have to have faith in what they've learned and the experience they have gained.

My greatest fear at this moment is that I've wasted time. As I write this book, I am fifty-five. By the time I quit squirreling around in my head and finish it, I'll be a smidge older. I don't necessarily believe that my time is running out, but I'm pretty sure I have less of it than I did when I discovered my gifts, and I have so much to share.

My health journey has been all over the place. I was an average child, a good athlete as a teenager, a hard-working twenty-year-old, a fitness-lazy thirty-year-old, an uber-fit forty-year-old, and a frustrated, depressed, ready-to-give-up fifty-year-old. I'm a certified nutritionist, personal trainer, and life coach, but I couldn't find my way to the ever-distant destination of sustainable health.

My past life established many good habits. I ate "healthy food" and knew the importance of exercise for muscle maintenance and stress relief. But it wasn't until I started focusing on enjoying delicious food, moving every day in ways that bring me joy, reading for pleasure, journaling regularly, viewing the world through a lens of gratitude, and making sleep a priority that my body started to change.

I've been a size 4, and I've been a size 20. I'm currently swinging back and forth between 12 and 14. I don't have a size goal; I have a "feel goal." I've prayed to feel good, and I'm getting there. I've prayed to feel beautiful. With help, encouragement, and the loving words of my husband and family, I do. I've prayed to live a good life in this good body that I've been gifted, and as I listen to my gut and my God, I've learned that it's not as hard as I've been making it.

Through a long series of events, I've lived the life of my dreams. I've known good people, and I've raised good people. I've worried about making ends meet, and I've had excess. I've been extraordinarily healthy, and I've been sick. I've worked hard and enjoyed traveling to many beautiful places. I ran a gym, coached thousands of people, gained life experience, and discovered that I am gloriously gifted in seeing the best in people. God put me on this planet so I can tell you how wonderful you are, and if you allow yourself to trust me, you'll start to see it, too.

I believe this now more than ever because I've started to see it in myself.

Now, a bit about this book:

- I organized the chapters in a way I hoped would work for all readers. Each of us is at a different place on our health journey, and as my friend Roberta reminded me, "People are only going to change one step at a time." You can fly through the first few chapters if you're an experienced journaler with a good self-image and a workout routine. But if you're just beginning your journey, you have my permission to take it slow. You have the rest of your life to achieve your goals- put a few habits in place along the way to ensure your hard work pays off and lasts forever.

- I wrote this book with a seven-week timeline in mind, so I divided the chapters into sections, imagining each as an encounter we might have on a given day at the gym. There is a lesson or a story that allows us a bit of time to interact, and then I send you on your way to work through habits on your own. Usually, the sections are short, so you can move through them one per day if you're in a hurry or bite off a more significant chunk if your schedule allows. Most of the time, I included prompts or questions. I encourage you to take things at your own pace. Wading In = small steps in a new direction. Deep Dive = life-changing work. Choose the ones that feel right and save the others for another day.
- I introduced you to a few people who helped me realize there were many paths to health. They made a forever imprint on my life and changed the way I approached my journey. I encourage you to find your own inspiration as you move through life.
- I included scripture and stories of how my expanding faith has made my journey more joy-filled.
- I referred you to excellent partners- people who have made it easier to feel good on the way to a healthier me. I encourage you to identify these people in your community and reach out to them sooner rather than later. My life could have been much easier if I'd sought help earlier.
- I included recipes, pantry lists, and ideas to make cooking fun in the "Back of the Book."
- Finally, I shared two habits that significantly impacted reversing my Deep Dive: **Learning to Listen** and **Crowding Out.** These two practices can be applied to any area of your

life you'd like to change. The questions at the end of each section will help you Learn to Listen, and I'll give you several examples of ways to Crowd Out at the end of each chapter.

Learning to Listen

If I've learned one thing in fifty-five years, it's that there is no right or wrong when it comes to living my best life. Some things worked for me when I was twenty. Many of those things don't work for me now. In the same respect, many of my current practices wouldn't fit in my life when I was younger.

Whether you're trying to revamp your diet, exercise routine, prayer, or social life, there isn't one right way. We've all seen today's miracle cure become tomorrow's nightmare too often to say there is only one way to become healthy.

So, what does this mean in a world of too much information and on-demand options?

I had to learn to listen to my body, and because I'm older and chronically distracted, I realized the need to write things down. "Listening" often means tracking a new supplement or exercise for a few days (or weeks) to see what manifests after I try something new.

Intuition is a powerful tool no matter what the task. Trust how you feel and work HARD to get back to a place where the voices in your head, the feelings of your heart, the hunger of your body, and the desires of your imagination originate from within you.

It might be the most challenging work you've ever done, but it's worth it to reset your operating system to get back to the way you were when you were born. You are meant to feel sensations like hunger or fatigue and respond in a particular way. You're also created to dream, explore, question, and live in community. I shared my stories and offered a nudge to get back to *you*.

I think it's also important to note that sustainable change is more likely if you approach your goals from a positive place. Your brain is more willing to follow your lead when it thinks you're going to do something fun. For example, if you set a positive goal, "I'm going to eat five servings of fruit or vegetables a day," you can feel good checking them off. If you set a deprivation goal, "I won't eat junk food," your brain kicks into the terrible-two-temper mode, demanding its needs be fulfilled. Set goals you feel good about and can reasonably expect to achieve.

Crowding Out

In theory, crowding out is the act of displacing one thing or action in favor of an option more aligned with your goals. The more new things you add, the less room you have for the old, allowing you to create new tastes or habits without feeling deprived.

Most of the time, when someone talks about "getting healthy," they share a complicated plan complete with a list of rules detailing calories, macros, exercise, sleep, meditation… on and on and on. They often describe the things they are going to give up rather than what they get to keep.

There is nothing I dislike more than someone telling me what to do. It started when I was young, and it continues today. Tell me I can't do something and watch me try…

Tell me I can't eat something, and watch me struggle with the cravings. Tell me I can't have wine and watch the final drops from the bottle trickle into my glass. Tell me I should exercise, and I'll find a new series to binge-watch. Sound familiar?

But what about if I order a salad as my side and barter a couple of fries from my husband? Or enjoy a glass of wine followed by a glass of water instead of automatically pouring *another* glass of wine? What if I take a long walk with a friend instead of texting back and forth for hours and let that count as my daily exercise?

Here's another example: there was a time in my life when I only drank coffee and sugared soda. I didn't drink water unless I had to take a pill or brush my teeth! I'd wake up in the morning, and my first priority was coffee. I'd often drink three or more big cups a day, each enhanced with cream and sugar. Once mid-morning rolled around, I'd switch over to soda. I worked in a restaurant, so it was readily available and free. After two or more throughout the day, I'd fill a 32-ounce cup before leaving work and sip on it all night.

When I became pregnant with my first son, I tried to cut the "bad things" out of my life, including caffeine. I quit drinking all of my regular beverages as soon as I found out I was expecting, but I experienced mood swings and horrible headaches almost immediately. I didn't want to take medication to alleviate the pain and quickly fell back into my caffeinated routine.

After a few days of feeling "normal," I tried again, weaning myself off caffeine by replacing my third coffee with water and reducing my evening soda. I allowed myself to sip on it until we finished dinner and then switched to water. The following week, I dropped another coffee and reduced the size of my soda again, each time adding a little more water. Following this "add in the good" plan, I cut caffeine from my diet and increased my water intake for four weeks with few adverse effects.

I was formally introduced to crowding out[2] when participating in the Institute of Integrative Nutrition's (IIN) Health Coach Training Program. In hindsight, I've been using it myself and in my nutrition coaching practice for many years.

I've discovered this method of adding in works for many other areas in my life. There are several examples of ways to crowd out habits that may be keeping you from your best life, without feeling deprived. Feel free to share ways you crowd out on your journey. I love learning new ways to keep me on the path towards my goals!

It's not my intention to label things as good and bad, but rather present you with food, drink, and lifestyle add-ins that have made my healthy lifestyle sustainable with less suffering!

♥

The Journey

Sitting on the runway with a ticket to paradise can be exciting. I try to pick the perfect destination outfit and to avoid being uncomfortable, I often end up lugging a carry-on full of things "just in case". The slippers and blankets seem like a great idea when I'm packing, but deciding what's important before I store my bag can be overwhelming. Nine times out of ten, I choose only my phone, a book, and a water bottle to get through the journey. Meanwhile, my purse is bursting at the seams, and I need my husband to help me get the luggage into the overhead bin because I've overpacked.

I struggle to enjoy the trip because I get caught up in the details. Turning your health around can feel like that, too.

I used to draw a line in the sand and make a plan. I'd circle a date on the calendar in red ink and tell myself, "This time, I'll finally reach the promised land, and it will be amazing." I'd fill my bag with rules and restrictions that worked in the past, forgetting that I wasn't the same woman I was in my twenties, and ignore the fact that that it didn't work back then either.

Once all of the preparations were in order, I did everything I could to put it off because I was afraid this time would be like all the others; I'd waste effort and money to get to my destination, but when I arrived, it wouldn't be the way I expected.

Have you ever felt like that?

What if, this time, you traveled on your terms?

What if I told you it's also okay to be who you are, where you are, and still want more? What if you packed only the basic things that that made you happy? And what if there was no named final destination? Oh! And what if the trip was all-inclusive and you had hundreds of options to make the journey your own?

This is what I'm offering you.

I included the chapters in the order I would prescribe and offered suggestions to incorporate some habits that have finally brought joy back into the journey for me. Try them one at a time, so you can ease into your new life.

Please try to fight the urge to read about food first. I know you because I am you, and I've skipped the first 50% of all the wellness books I've purchased just to get to the "good stuff." Indulge me for a short time, if you will, please.

"A journey of a thousand miles begins with a single step," so trust me for just a little while. The small steps I suggest might help you finally find your path to joy and self-love on your journey to better health.

Recording. Knowing your goals. Moving your body. They are all essential steps before you start to change your diet. Too often, we get stuck in our past, believing the only way is the "old way," and we starve ourselves to see changes.

If your goals are the same as twenty years ago, you're not being fair to yourself. If you slash your calories to lose weight while sitting on the couch every day, you're not being fair, either. You need fewer calories to sit than you do if you're moving. Move your body first, and learn to eat when you're hungry. It's good to be hungry, even better when you learn to satisfy that hunger in ways that help you live a long, joy-filled life.

I'm a woman with a degree in life. I have plenty of certifications and bucketloads of experience. I've struggled for a long time to love myself, but I've finally arrived at a place of graceful acceptance. I had to learn it's okay to be who I am and still want something different.

The words on the following pages come from my heart and hopefully reflect a new way of looking at life. I want to share the joy I experience every day. I hope you find a way to read a little each day, gathering the pieces you need to make your return to health a journey that lasts a lifetime.

♥

Chapter 1

Give it Up

Faith Journey

So, where does faith fit in a health book? I've been trying to tie it together for a while, and after battling the pounds the traditional way ever since my gym closed, it dawned on me how many times I've fallen back into gimmick diets, cleanses, and high-impact cardio.

I'd promise to behave, deprive myself of everything delicious, vow not to drink another glass of wine, and force myself to walk at a stupid pace, on an incline, in a place that smells like an old shoe.

The difference this time is the lens in which I'm viewing myself:

- I'm no longer dieting because I want to be thinner; I'm choosing foods because I want to feel good.
- I'm no longer exercising to burn calories; I'm moving to gain strength and flexibility.
- I'm no longer hiding from the camera; I'm engaging in a life worth sharing.
- I'm no longer saving my story; I'm sharing it to help someone else.
- I'm no longer telling myself, "someday." Today is the day given to me, and there may not be another. And today, I am worthy, I am beautiful, and I am loved.

My purpose this time isn't simply to look better. It's longevity, legacy, and mission-driven. And although my Creator finds joy when I appreciate the gifts He's given me, I believe He's setting me up for something greater than I've accomplished thus far.

I was writing in my journal one morning, making yet another "I'll start Monday" promise to myself, and as I turned the page to continue, I noticed the words printed on the bottom of the blank sheet:

"You are altogether beautiful, my love;
there is no flaw in you."

Song of Solomon 4:7

The tears started flowing, and I wasn't quite sure why. At my age, in my current hormonal condition, I cry pretty often! I wrapped up my journaling and headed outdoors for a walk, but I couldn't shake the scripture or my reaction.

Was it random timing, or were the words placed there for me when I needed them most? The coincidence was interesting, considering the written lashing I was giving myself moments before turning the page. Throughout my walk, it occurred to me how horribly I treat myself when I "fail." I say things to myself I would never say to a client.

I rarely walk with music in my ears because I like to be aware of my surroundings. I prefer walking alone in the morning and use this quiet time to work through things. It was a beautiful blue sky kind of day. The trees in full foliage and the wind moving through sounded like rushing water. I thought how good it must feel to create something so wonderful....

Then the realization came- I am one of His creations, unique and special in many ways. My size is simply one part of who I am, and hiding myself until I am "just right" denies the artist His due.

I am loved. I am loved by my husband, my sons and their wives, my parents, and so many others. I am loved by my Creator. I've always been loved, from the moment I was created in my mother's womb to the here and now... I am loved.

Even today, as I write this, I have to admit I fall back. There are days when I feel alone and ugly based on earthly standards. Days when I don't want to leave the house because my pants don't fit or because there might be someone at an event who "knew me when." It's at these moments, it's most important to remind myself I am wonderfully made and loved, just as I am.

My faith journey started long ago when I was a little girl. We didn't go to church much, but I remember saying bedtime prayers with my mom:

"Now I lay me down to sleep,
I pray the Lord my soul to keep.
If I should die before I wake,
I pray the Lord my soul to take." [1]

Follow that bit of childhood memory with God bless Mommy and Daddy and every other person I knew. Some nights, my blessing list would go on and on (and on) to delay actual bedtime.

My next distinct memory was Vacation Bible School. It was held up the road from our house in a church we didn't attend regularly. I got to go because my sister was born that summer, and I'm sure Mom just needed a break from her constantly questioning four-year-old. At VBS, I learned another oldie but goodie, "Here is the church, here is the steeple..." I remember practicing in the back seat of the car so I could show my grandparents! So exciting!

That was the extent of my church life until junior high. We didn't go to church, but somehow, we must have "lived" church because I remember feeling like God was a big deal. I remember searching the December sky for the star that led the wise men to the baby Jesus, and I remember praying to Him when our home seemed out of control.

Junior High brought about a lot of changes in my world. My parents were not getting along. They separated for some time, and when my dad quit drinking, Mom let him move back in. Life was super cool for a while, like, so amazing I thought God answered all my prayers, and we would live happily ever after as a family of four. We talked at the dinner table, Dad helped with homework, and he went with us to swim meets. Basic family outings became special events simply because they had never happened before.

Work stress and untreated coping habits eventually led Dad to buy a six-pack, which turned into much more over the months to come, and my mom filed for divorce. He moved seventeen hours away, and suddenly, Mom decided we should go to church. There is probably more to it, but that's what I remember (and if I ever go to therapy, there is a bucket load of things I need to work out before I get to that!).

I loved attending church and dove head first into everything, like confirmation class and choir. I met new friends and eventually joined the youth group. Confirmation was led by the senior pastor, who was a good man and a good preacher. I learned things I didn't know, which was important.

Youth group was the bomb! It was led by the associate pastor named Jerry. He lived in the parsonage next door to the church and was so good about planning activities that let us all be together. We went horseback riding, raked leaves, and baked bread at his house. I don't remember discussing scripture, but I certainly remember feeling loved and, more importantly, feeling like I was a part of something good.

Mom remarried a few years later, and we moved a couple of hours away from that church, but I've never forgotten the people who helped with the earliest formation of my faith.

I thought all of the good things I would ever experience were in my hometown, and I turned into a bit of a demon when Mom decided to uproot our happy little family. I'm not terribly proud of that time. I was lippy and absent and determined to make her pay.

We joined a new church where she had taken a job as an administrative coordinator. We attended regularly as a family, but in hindsight, she probably would have preferred I stay home. I made it my mission to pull scripture out of context to use against people who thought differently than I did. I'd still stand behind the reasons I did so, but as a more mature Christian, I dislike it very much when people isolate a few words to shove an opinion down the throat of someone else.

I took a break from all things church after high school, citing work and school as my main excuses. In my hiatus, I still believed in God. I just wasn't sure if He believed in me.

In the meantime, I started college, quit college, and accepted a full-time job. Before I knew it, I fell in love.

We were married in my parents' church, and just a few short months later, I discovered I was pregnant. My friends, that was it for me. The miracle of the life inside me turned me to prayer over and over again (in all honesty, those prayers were often on my knees in the bathroom for the first four months). I was young and so in love with the creature twisting and turning inside of me. I may have been a skeptic before, but in those early months of my twenty-first year, I came to believe in all God can do. I had never felt so blessed or so in love.

Zachary was born three days after our first anniversary. My son was a gift. He was healthy, happy, and content almost all the time! I felt like I was finally doing the one thing I was meant to do, and he was such a good baby. It was easy to assume life would always be easy.

The early years of motherhood flew by in a blur. As young parents, we worked a lot and often manipulated our schedules so one of us could be home with Zach. Late-night shifts and money fights got in the way of the good times, and I once again forgot that I could turn to God for anything. My marriage fell apart. I could blame a hundred different things, but as I sit here, thirty years later, I can only blame the lack of good role models, my lack of commitment, and our inability to communicate.

I remarried a few years later, and after some time, we decided to have another child. I was pregnant within months, and again, I realized there was something incredible about carrying life within me, and not surprisingly, my faith was rekindled.

Samuel was born on a cold December night. He was a month early but seemingly perfect at first breath. However, his health turned at an alarming rate. Within minutes, he was whisked away from our hospital room to the NICU for evaluation. Our youngest son was in critical condition, requiring three blood transfusions over several days to compensate for his critically low hemoglobin. The doctors hoped to "jump start" his body into producing red blood cells. I prayed more than I've ever prayed before. My husband prayed. Our families prayed, and my mom's church prayed. Everyone prayed.

We walked out of the hospital ten days after he was born, thanks to doctors and nurses and one donor who gifted us with enough plasma to give my tiny son the time he needed to heal.

Our little boy grew and thrived with no apparent consequences. And we gave thanks.

My next spirit-lead encounter occurred at his six-month check-up. His pediatrician swept into the exam room, excited to share that he had presented Sam's case to his peers just the day before.

Hmm. Why is that?

I learned that day that most children born with his complications didn't survive unscathed- in fact, he may have been one of the first infants to survive and thrive.

My thankfulness grew! My faith grew! God had given me my own little miracle. And I owed Him so much!

I dove into church like it was my regular job. I worked in child care as a Sunday school teacher and coordinated the yearly Advent festival. I joined classes, and I studied at home. I sat in church, wept during baptisms, and sensed the light beams filtering through the stained glass windows were signs just for me.

As a twenty-nine-year-old stay-at-home mother of two, I found myself lonely and looking for friends. My husband worked long hours, and in my service at church, I fell into a comfortable rhythm of conversation with a young pastor. She was kind and reflective. Listening to her speak was like listening to the ancient wisdom of the great women of the Bible, and I was so enamored by her. I read books and joined study groups at her suggestion. On the third Thursday of each month, I bared my soul to a room full of women gathered for a small group. I made new friends and felt like I had found my place. I loved being a good Christian woman: reflecting, being artistic and honest, sharing my Jesus story with them.

Then, one night, the woman I had promoted to high priestess revealed she was, in fact, a flesh and blood human. She was upset about something that happened in her "real life ."She unknowingly said things to a room full of women that felt directed at me. The words hurt me and pulled out my deep, hidden feelings of unworthiness, burning holes into my uneducated, "just a mom" heart. I left that night ashamed at the thought I could ever be good enough to belong.

I never returned and didn't tell her how her words made me feel. I think I left God behind that night as well. I closed off everything holy and refused to let myself be vulnerable again.

Fast forward many years… lost years when my sons were not exposed to God regularly. The boys knew we believed, but they grew up with theories and opinions rather than traditions and truth. We lived in a house of "Jesus -my way," or conditional faith, using the stories and teachings that felt right while leaving several tough truths behind. Not surprisingly, we had a hard time finding a place to worship that spoke to us all.

I lost my in-laws and my grandmother during those years. My nephew had a life-altering accident as well. God reached out to me each time through people or memories. He tried again and again to comfort me, but I barely acknowledged His existence, let alone His love.

I achieved business success at this time as well. I did good things for people, so in my mind, I was a good person. I achieved everything I ever wanted in my professional career, but I was absent at home and on the verge of losing everything that mattered.

Sometime as I neared my fiftieth birthday, my heart started stirring again. I began by reading a book here or there, especially around the major Christian holidays, and then branched off into "write the word" journals during my early morning quiet time. I enjoyed learning more about God, but I still wasn't talking to Him and certainly wasn't listening.

March 2020 arrived, and we all know what happened. The pandemic caused me to step up my game (just in case, you know?). I'm sure I'm not the only one who called Him up out of the blue. Can you imagine how the lines to heaven jammed up that year?

Fortunately, I never heard, "I'm sorry, please hold."

He was right there, once again, waiting for me to return.

I fell into a routine of watching church on YouTube. I chose a specific church because many of my family members attended services there. There was a connection, and they were already up and running online when I figured out I needed church most.

Side note: I teased my mother-in-law for watching TV preachers when she was still earthbound. I bet she and God got a good chuckle out of me sipping coffee in my bathrobe on Sunday mornings, singing out loud, and crying over a sermon or two!

Eventually, our state lessened restrictions, and the local site of the same church started having services in a park in my hometown. I considered attending a few times but kept settling into my comfy chair on Sunday mornings. I guess I figured I was still okay on my own. The world hadn't ended; God was present in my life, and I was diving into the word more than ever.

In time, my son's fiancee asked me to attend a service with her. She heard the young pastor was a gifted preacher, and she and Sam were looking for a church home. We headed out on a brisk Sunday morning, still in masks, and set our chairs up far outside the gathering space so no one would recognize us. I didn't want to feel pressured to return if I wasn't comfortable.

The leaves were changing, the wind was blowing, the music was incredible, and the dear Lord placed the words I needed to hear on the lips of that young pastor that day.

I returned time and time again, each time receiving something I needed. Sometimes, it was a song, sometimes scripture, sometimes the message, but always the feeling.

I've never experienced church like that before; I was in awe of the faith I saw around me and the Spirit I felt in my heart. I encountered people who simply loved Jesus. No rules, no restrictions. Just open, honest, and caring people focused on building community and sharing His love. I encountered people who live the Word rather than simply speaking it.

It's occurred to me over the last few years that faith is like everything else. Just like there isn't a perfect diet or workout, there isn't a perfect way to worship. Like all of the other good things in life, you have to find your way to God in a way that feels right to you.

When I'm gone, someone will have the opportunity to read my most private thoughts from the journals hidden strategically in my home, and they'll undoubtedly realize they didn't know me at all.

I put on a happy face, and I try to see the best in everyone. I act like I have my life together and I've figured out my way. But throughout the pages where I allow my heart to wander, I explore the moments when I felt far from God. In my early journals, one will find list after list after list of should haves, could haves, and what-ifs. And after each of those lists, there is the obligatory self-shaming session where I attempt to justify my desires despite my blessings:

How is it that I could receive so much and yet still feel unsatisfied?

Can I be thankful and still want more?

Can I be angry? Can I feel alone?

Will He love me if I walk away for a time?

The answer, again and again, is yes.

God wants us to prosper. He wants us to be happy, healthy, and satisfied, but in our rush to do everything, acquire everything, and BE all things, we have forgotten how to be thankful.

Throughout this chapter, I'll share a few practices that have helped me shift my posture from desire to gratitude. As I work to reconcile my relationship with God, my expectations have changed. I've accepted His love and grace, which are never-ending, and learned that He wants me to be happy. Through this, I've begun to notice things that bring me undeniable joy.

My list of blessings continues to grow.

Wading In: List three things that made you happy today.

Deep Dive: Count your blessings~ one for every year you've been alive.
I challenge you to be specific.

My 55th Birthday list is in the "Back of the Book" if you get stuck and want some ideas.

♥

Be Careful

It's interesting that we (middle-aged Americans) spend our lives working to acquire the best things... the best clothes, the best education, the best partner. We mortgage our lives to drive the best car to the best home in the best school district to take pictures with the best cell phone and share them with the world.

But what happens when you finally reach your financial goals and have time to contemplate your life? Do you like the person you chose to spend your life with? Do you like the people you made? Do you play catch with the dog you had to have? Do you take off your shoes and walk in the grass you paid to grow? Do you turn off the lights and look at the stars? Do you wake up early, open the blinds, and watch the sunrise?

Today, I had the good fortune to wake up 1,500 miles from home. I opened my eyes, adjusted to the dark, and planned my day from the comfort of bed.

"Sunrise is at 7:11, so I need to be out the door by 6:40 to catch the best colors, leaving me time to dress, drink coffee, journal, and pray before I go."

I slid out of bed quietly, padding down the stairs to make coffee. I grabbed a glass of water and settled in with my journal, finishing my entry with plenty of time to spare. Then, I remembered my coffee, and I hadn't dressed for my walk yet, and somehow, it was already 6:38.

My schedule feels funky. I'm trying new things for the first time in two years, and I keep forgetting what I'm supposed to do. I took a moment to sip some lukewarm coffee and dashed up the stairs to change clothes. Thankfully, they were set out the night before. I was up and down in no time. I tied my tennies and rushed out the door three minutes behind schedule.

The beach was deserted. It was the first workday of the new year. There was a lone fisherman to the south, and I turned that direction to keep the sunrise in front of me. It's too easy to forget to turn around once I get to the shell-embedded dunes. Without words or music, I walk in the pre-dawn light, watching the waves crash into the shore. I made it past the fisherman without a sound. He was focused on his empty hook, and I was searching for a hag stone to send to my stepmom. I looked up to check the sun and almost ran into a fully-grown crane! She was staring intently at me, and I'm sure she was wondering if I would stop or completely bowl her over in my quest for the perfect rock.

I was startled and hopped back a bit. She tilted her head as if to say hello. And then majestically strolled to the water's edge. She stood knee-deep in the waves, watching the sunrise.

We prayed together that morning. She, with her silent attention, and I on my knees on the dune, surrounded by broken shells and driftwood. Little birds twittered around her, yet she stood, unwavering, watching the sun. Two different creatures, the crane and I… unable to communicate, but both in awe of all He provides.

Suddenly, a feathered friend distracted her, and they set off on a bit of a chase. I rose from my knees, gathered my belongings, and started back up the beach. After all this time, the only other human on the beach was still the fisherman I'd passed earlier, tending his line.

Beautiful homes line the beach, high-rise condos and sprawling mansions. The best that money can buy, yet I was alone, with the fisherman and the crane, to witness the most glorious show of the day.

More than ever, our society seems dissatisfied, depressed, angry, and sick because we have forgotten to appreciate what is good, beautiful, and free to experience. We neglect our creative souls, forgetting to enjoy as we set impossible goals, trudging through forty years or more with our heads down. Moving ahead without looking up. Checking off the list without saying thanks. Pretending that we created this life and never take the time to enjoy it.

What happened to us? Didn't we all reach adulthood with hopes and dreams? How did we get so caught up in a life full of checklists and expectations?

I am the biological daughter of a perfectionist and a caretaker. The best I can figure is that this combination made me feel like I could never be good enough, but with hard work and love, I would likely be okay. As I reflect on my first fifty years, I realize how feeling like I was "not enough" pushed me to be impulsive and in-your-face when people didn't agree with me. I've created most of the conflict in my life by not relinquishing control.

"I can do better than anyone!" was my battle cry.

Maybe I did for a while until I burnt out, got bored, or chased off everyone who mattered in my world.

Doing better, a.k.a. creating the world I prayed for, created much heartache, and as a result, I found myself teetering on the edge of self-destruction. I had everything I wanted but had fallen into a routine of neglecting the things I needed.

Writing this book has caused some of these feelings to resurface. I have a million great ideas, but the words don't write themselves. It's easy to get caught up in moments of self-doubt. I sit at my computer some mornings, fingers seemingly paralyzed by the fear that my story is just my story and no one really cares.

Through the conversations of a tight-knit writers cohort, I've learned this is called Imposter Syndrome. It's a psychological occurrence in which an individual doubts their skills, talents, or accomplishments and has a persistent internalized fear of being exposed as a fraud.

Add this self-imposed affliction to my pre-existing feelings of inadequacy, and I can experience writer's block for several days. A brilliant idea will pop into my head, and within moments, it becomes drivel, landing on the page in a mess that doesn't make sense. I struggle with what is relevant and what is simply filler. A million ideas. Which should I write about first?

I've been stuck this week, but today, mid-shower, as the shampoo was running down the drain, my fog lifted, and I realized how well my ideas work together.

I repeatedly heard, "Be careful what you pray for…"

In all of my hardest times, I prayed for what I wanted, and when my answer didn't come the way I wanted, I made it happen myself.

"I'll show you," surfaced again and again as I rushed into so many life-altering moments. I've depleted my savings and wasted time I should have spent with my boys. I pushed my husband away when his help and guidance could have made many things better and more sustainable.

As I dive deeper into my relationship with God, I find myself trying to listen, which requires so much patience. Of all my skills, listening, followed by patience, are the ones I need to work on the most.

I think about the life-changing moments that could have gone differently:

Teenage rebellion

Quitting college

Marriage

Divorce

Quitting my job

Opening a business

Closing a business

The list goes on and on and on. I know God was always with me, but I'm pretty sure I had my earbuds in to drown out His whispers of patience, common sense, and purpose.

What if I would have prayed for clarity and waited? Or if I would have prayed for counsel and listened? Would I be in a different place today?

I believe I did good things, but I also know I could have done better if I'd stashed my ambition and pride in the trunk, allowing the Spirit to drive while I rode shotgun once in a while.

I'm trying to be more mindful of what I pray for; I still ask for things I want, but I've tried to open my heart, asking for guidance and patience when I receive the answers I didn't expect.

Wading In: Do you have unanswered prayers?

Deep Dive: Explore an answer you weren't expecting.

♥

Childlike Faith

At that time the disciples came to Jesus, saying, "Who is the greatest in the kingdom of heaven?" And calling to him a child, he put him in the midst of them and said, "Truly, I say to you, unless you turn and become like children, you will never enter the kingdom of heaven."

Matthew 18:1-3

In every crowded room, whether full of strangers or friends, you will find someone you're drawn to. You might have similar interests or acquaintances, or maybe it's how they interact with others… smiling, open, and engaged.

I met thousands of incredible people at my gym. Some of them have become lifelong friends through the intertwining of our stories.

I met one such person through a group who had transferred from another gym when I first opened. She wasn't a challenger; she slipped into membership through the "past experience loophole."

Jennifer was quiet. She never actively pursued people but drew them in like the light beckoning moths at twilight. She was glowing, warm, and available. Before class, she would talk with one or two friends, sharing stories about their day. People would wander into the conversation, and she always engaged them with questions, truly caring what they had to say.

As the years passed, she included me in her circle, greeting me and sharing joys and significant life events, but it always felt like she was keeping a part of her story to herself. By how she interacted with people, I guessed she had once been the moth drawn to a bright light that eventually burnt her. I'd often see her smile twist as someone said just the right (wrong?) thing. The fire in her eyes would dim briefly as she wandered to a place of memories.

It wasn't until several years into our relationship that she let me all the way in. At the time, she was pregnant and curious about her health and wellness in a new way. She and her husband had battled with infertility, and she was adamant that she cared for the new life that had finally taken hold within her womb in the best way possible.

She's since had another child, and I've been blessed to be included in her life, watching her grow as she evolves in her role as a mother.

One day, she reached out with a question that wasn't about nutrition; it was about my faith. Her church and Bible experience were limited, which surprised me because I'd always noticed her faith was great. I learned that she realized her need for Jesus while going through the ups and downs of trying to conceive. At her last straw and desperate for help, she turned to prayer, begging a loving God to bless her with her heart's desire.

She is an avid learner and has become an unashamed worshiper, moving to the music, sharing her story, volunteering in children's programs, and selflessly praying for others. She can find Jesus in the most unexpected places. Surprisingly, she sees His work in me.

I've read the Bible a few times in my life. Until recently, I've interpreted it from the viewpoint of historical fiction, considering it to be stories passed through the generations to explain an event in time. I've been known to say things like, "Don't take the story so literally… this was an unscientific telling by someone with minimal knowledge of the world".

I've often approached her questions from that perspective, reassuring her that a particular verse doesn't apply today. It's simply meant to remind us where we came from. Fortunately, my friend is insistent. She reads carefully and thinks thoroughly, circling back to conversations when she's unsatisfied with my answer.

Jennifer has pushed me, more times than she knows, to blow the dust off the scripture I've memorized to search for the story that will move me today. She shares songs and podcasts, sometimes daily, pushing me to explore points of view I might never stumble across without her.

And though not a child, her faith is childlike. She's hungry for knowledge, wants to be obedient, and is faithful, never doubting His grace. Her pursuit of Him has made me rethink my own journey. What is different about us?

I take classes. I attend worship and sing loudly (my heartfelt apology to you if you've ever stood in front of me). I volunteer. I've embraced a posture of gratitude. All of these are good and faithful actions, but there's one thing that keeps me from living my life as a child of God.

Through all I've done, I've never, for one second, given up control. My actions may have drawn me closer to Him, but I have difficulty releasing my grip on my life.

On the other hand, she is content to depend on God to provide for her needs and protect her from harm. She trusts her prayers will be answered. She believes in His never-ending love.

As I attempt to release my need to control everything in my life, I've tried to view my practices through the eyes of one new to faith. I've begun to incorporate some childlike practices into my routine:

- **Pray every day and for anything**
- **Spend time outside playing (borrow a kid if you need an excuse to swing)**
- **Love without qualification**

- **Be excited about your gifts and express your thanks formally (Be the best at snail mail thank you cards!)**
- **Give gifts to others (even if the only thing on hand is a bright yellow dandelion)**
- **Do new things**
- **Say you're sorry when you hurt someone**
- **Forgive when someone hurts your feelings**
- **Trust that you are loved, and nothing will take that away**

My friend showed me the difference between knowing the word of God and believing in His promises. She taught me the difference between memorizing scripture and remembering the stories of the ones who came before us. And she's modeled over and over again what it looks like to place faith in my Creator rather than trying to control my destiny alone.

Wading In: How can you be more childlike?

Deep Dive: What could you give up to live as a child of God?

♥

Take Delight

"Take delight in the Lord, and he will give you your heart's desires."

Psalm 37:4

Today, I was walking to the beach, planning to look for shells while waiting for the sun to rise. This has become my routine: wake, write, walk, watch the sunrise, and chat with God.

If I diagrammed those early morning conversations, I would likely see that I do a lot of the talking. I often ask for help, especially during the hard times, and I try to say thank you. Unfortunately, I've spent very little time listening.

We seem to have our best conversations when I'm not distracted by shells, so I was thankful for a day when the beach was wiped clean of treasures. The water roared and crashed around me, and I asked for inspiration. Waves carried spirals of broken shells that looked like calla lilies, and I stashed a few in my bag, each filling a vase in my imagination. I offered thanks for each treasure but spent most of the morning wrestling with the thoughts bouncing around in my head.

As I neared my turnaround point, I saw a large object sitting alone on the beach just out of the reach of the waves. My pace quickened a bit, hoping it was more than a waterlogged coconut. I was rewarded with a glorious blue-gray whelk, larger than my foot and in excellent condition; I turned it over and over in my hands. It was stunning! I tried to imagine the creature that once lived inside and the pride I would feel if I had created this home. I felt rewarded and inspired!

My random thoughts calmed, and I heard instead, "You can be broken and empty, but you can still bring great joy. Your original purpose may be through, but you can become something new".

It occurred to me that maybe, just maybe, God looks at me the way I've been viewing the shells every morning. Perhaps he sees the beauty in the spiral of my insides. Maybe he finds joy in thinking about where I've been. Maybe he imagines what I can be now that I've raised my sons and retired from my career.

Maybe He pauses to say thanks for me.

Once I started considering my unfailing worth in His eyes, I found it easier to view God as my confidant and a trusted friend. Often, I talk to Him in the most informal way; I might start a prayer with "Hey God" or "Hello again." Sometimes, it's as simple as touching a shell or smelling a flower and whispering, "Thank you."

I imagine the loneliness He might feel when he offers amazing gifts, and we don't notice. A world that can't slow to stand in awe at sunset or pause to watch an eclipse will rarely find joy in smaller things like the smell of fresh-cut grass, the taste of a perfect berry, or the smile of a stranger.

Some might shudder at the informal posture I take with God. I've spent hundreds of anxious moments worrying about it myself. When it comes to prayer, am I doing it right?

Do I offend when I speak informally or hurt His feelings when I am too preoccupied to experience the gifts all around?

Is it okay to turn to memorized prayers or read someone else's words?

Does He understand when I have no choice but to stand in silence, allowing my emotions to take over when words won't form?

Will He help me overcome my fear to pray out loud at the dinner table or in front of others (especially if they know more theology than I do)?

Again and again, I believe the answer to every question is yes.

Fortunately, I put my faith in a God who has faith in me. He keeps offering me opportunities, and I want to share them with you.

Angel Numbers

About a year ago, I started noticing recurring numbers, like 11:11 or 4:44. I typed "What does it mean if I keep seeing the number 11:11" into my favorite search engine and read more than I wanted to know about numerology. I learned these numbers can have many meanings. I was intrigued by the message behind some of them, but it also felt weird, so I abandoned my research and moved on.

Day after day, I kept seeing these number sequences, so many that I started to feel like someone was dangling a carrot. Eventually, I bit and decided to turn the regular occurrences into an opportunity to talk to God. I consider 12:12 or 5:55 a nudge from Him, a touch letting me know He's thinking about me.

Whenever I see the numbers, I stop what I'm doing and talk to my closest friend and confidant. Sometimes, it's as simple as "Hi, God! Thanks for reaching out. You must have known I was stressed and needed someone to talk to…" Other times when I feel like it's been too long, I'll devote more than a minute or two so I can dive in deep with a more formal prayer following A.C.T.S. (more on this in a second)

I love how I feel remembered, like He is a friend reaching out to check in with me, One who wants to know about my day. When I'm alone, I talk out loud to get used to using my voice when I pray.

A.C.T.S.

I try to be focused when I'm praying, but most mornings, my prayers are as interrupted as a feature film being played on basic cable with lots of commercial breaks. I often end up apologizing repeatedly for my sporadic nature, but breaking my prayer into parts has given me a little more structure. I learned about this type of prayer from other participants in my church's Intro to Prayer class. The following was one morning, one prayer, started and stopped five or more times:

Prayer of Adoration~ Honor Him: It's easy for me to start my morning prayer the moment I walk outside. I feel closest to God when I'm in nature, and I'm in awe of the littlest things:

"Oh, God. You are so good."

I walk for a while, taking it all in… bumble bees, light bouncing off the water, the details of a shell.

"Master artist. Perfect creator."

Prayer of Contrition~ Ask for forgiveness: As my steps fall into a rhythm, it's easy to reflect on my shortcomings:

"Please forgive me. I know I was wrong yesterday. I interrupted, needing to be right… wanting to be heard. I caused heartache and frustration at a time when I could have offered a listening ear and a place of comfort."

Prayer of Thanks~ Acknowledge the good in your life: I have many opportunities on any given day to give thanks, starting the moment I wake up! As a sensory person, I'm highly aware of sights, smells, sounds, and their absence. I try to offer gratitude when something strikes me as a gift or a prayer is answered.

Yesterday, I experienced the most incredible morning after a night of unsettled sleep. I had to make difficult decision and was thankful to walk out onto an empty beach rather than one full of treasures (shells) like the day before.

"Thank you for this morning. Thank you for a beach that's been washed clean of distraction. Thank you for the sunrise that causes me to pause, taking in the rolling waves. They remind me of your power that lies beyond my grasp."

Prayer of Supplication~ Ask for help: Because I walked on a beach void of shells, I had time to get lost in my thoughts, struggling with a decision.

"Help me to make this day productive, purposeful, and full of love. Help me to make the decisions I need to move my project forward and to remember my desires are not always the best for everyone."

Rarely do I let on to anyone that I don't know the answer to something, but since He already knows my struggles, I figured it was worth a shot. Within minutes, my answer came in the form of a perfect, beautiful shell lying in my path. It was unbroken and large enough to be considered a prize but not so big as for me to become distracted.

The answer formed in my mind, and for some reason, I spoke aloud:

"Help me make the choice that best represents my experience. The one that shares my simplest encounters so someone else might find joy and learn that You have no expectations when it comes to our love. Your love is unconditional and absolute. It's everywhere, and it's every day."

And as I stopped to repeat those words, to scorch them into memory, a wave crashed at my feet, carrying yet another perfectly formed shell.

"I love you... Thank you for loving me. Amen."

Intercessory Prayer

In the book *Prayer: Finding the Heart's True Home,* Richard J. Foster writes, "If we truly love people, we will desire for them far more than it is within our power to give them, and this will lead us to prayer. Intercession is a way of loving others."[2]

It is simply asking God's goodness and power to come into another person's life to provide healing or comfort.

Gone are the days when "God bless mommy and daddy and..." will suffice for me. It was a lovely start, but my requests have grown as I've experienced the power of prayer in my own life. It's easy to say, "I'll pray for you," but I wonder how many people follow through with words on another's behalf. I often approached the Father with requests when someone close to me was ill or hurt, but I've started to expand my list to include a few unsuspecting individuals who might not think they are in need. It's only recently that I've thought to reflect on the small miracles that are undoubtedly the result of another's prayers on my behalf. Thank heaven for those who pray!

I try to offer detailed prayers rather than summary prayers to "bless everybody." I know God knows everything, but I find keeping someone in my heart easier when I offer specific requests. As I get older, a prayer list in my journal helps me remember the details.

I also pray for God to reveal ways to help when I can. My answer is often to prepare a meal, but cards, calls, and visits also seem to suffice.

Prayer Journaling

I love to write and have been journaling regularly for quite some time, but I hadn't considered writing my prayers until I took a class last fall based loosely on the book *Let Prayer Change Your Life* by Becky Tirabassi[3]. In her book, the author shares her decision to pray for one hour a day and the result of her discipline. The benefits she describes are fascinating, but I couldn't imagine spending that much time writing in my journal, knowing I had other responsibilities as well.

During the first week of class, I set a goal of two pages of written prayer each day, but I struggled to make it different from the morning pages I was already writing. One day, I was so frustrated with my lack of ability that I set a timer for one minute to empty my mind and refocus. As the alarm chime notified me that time was up, I reset my timer for ten minutes. Miraculously, I turned to the pages, and the words flowed. Something about my session being time-bound freed my heart to allow the words to pour forth. I was mid-sentence when the timer went off again so soon! I've continued to lengthen the time as the months have passed. Who knows, maybe an hour is within reach!

Wading In: Make a list of people to pray for.

Deep Dive: How can I pray for you?

♥

Do Nothing

"Don't underestimate the value of doing nothing."

-A.A.Milne[4]

My people like noise. My husband and sons are very social beings who love music and activity. They play music when they work, listen to talk radio when they drive, and leave a TV on for background noise.

It makes me crazy.

There is nothing I crave more than silence. Not the sound booth variety, but the human distraction type of noise. I love long walks, listening to the wind move through the trees or the ocean crash upon the shore.

I can get lost in the absence of noise, allowing the thoughts in my head to wander until they find a central location to gather together and create beautiful things.

This silence hasn't always been easy.

I've tried to meditate countless times, usually coming out of a session with a fully formed grocery list and a few recipe ideas.

I've tried yoga, attempting to lose my thoughts in graceful movement. Still, it makes me anxious and sore, and I feel sorry for the person I'm likely distracting with my modified contortions. I've been told no one notices, but my insecurities tell me I will be featured on a remake of America's Funniest Home Videos.

I tried guided prayer using an app on my phone but got hung up on the recorded voice.

Finally, after taking the Intro to Prayer class at church and listening to experienced prayer partners share their stories, I tried several methods of centering prayer and landed on a technique that works for me.

Like with journaling, it turns out I need a timer to shut down my thoughts. It's like a backup that prevents my mind from wandering or worrying about tasks that will come later in the day.

I started with one minute, but that wasn't enough time to stop the eighty miles-per-hour progression of things in my head. So I set my timer for five minutes, repeated a single word, and with intentional breath, I could move into a state of nothingness as my mind slowed. I've come to moments of great clarity using this method of silence.

The practice reminds me of the controlled breathing I learned during Lamaze class as I prepared for my first son's birth. I've relied on this focused practice on many occasions since that intended day to manage pain, anxiety, and fear. For pain control, I combine it with a specific album of piano sonatas when undergoing "uncomfortable procedures." I don't like the long-term feeling of some pain medicines, and this practice has carried me through on several occasions with minimal medication.

I've always found it empowering to control my body and, recently, my mind. My prayer life is more focused and definitely more fruitful when I center myself, waiting for inspiration or direction.

Recently, I learned about *Breath Prayer*[5], breathing in at the top of a verse and exhaling at the bottom. It's a nice transition to the quiet I crave and it doesn't take long to still my mind if I use familiar text:

IN	OUT
Holy Spirit	Guide me (*John 16:13)*
I will not be afraid	For you are with me (*Psalm 23)*
The Lord is God	I am yours (*Psalm 100:3)*

And, if you feel rushed or anxious, try box breathing first to reach the place where you can silence your mind.

1. Close your eyes.
2. Count to four slowly on the inhale, visualizing a line moving from left to right.
3. Hold your breath, count to four slowly, and imagine drawing a line moving down the right side of a box.
4. Again, count to four slowly, exhaling as you move across the bottom of a square from right to left.
5. And hold, moving up the left side for a count of four.

Wading In: Practice Box Breathing before a busy time. Did it help?

Deep Dive: Set a timer for five minutes and empty your mind. What do you hear?

♥

Spirit Lead

My relationship with God is one of the most important things in my life, but it's also something I've often taken for granted or slipped on a shelf like a well-worn book when things are going well. It's easy to neglect those who love you unconditionally. The song may say you always hurt the one you love, and I think it's pretty easy to assume most of us take the One who loves us most for granted.

It's never been difficult for me to get into a routine of attending church on Sunday mornings. I look forward to worship, but it's pretty easy to slip right back into the drone of my everyday existence once the hour has passed. Life is busy, and there are visible distractions and obligations pulling at me every waking minute of the day. But as I'm trying to change my life and focus on what brings me joy, I'm deliberately trying to carry the Sunday message into my week.

If you're like I am, you would love to be in a deeper relationship with God and spend more time learning about his plan for your life, but it's hard to discern whether or not the call you hear is your voice or God's.

My church provides countless opportunities for extra learning and small group relationships, but there are moments when I'm in the middle of a group, and the words of my heart seem too personal or raw to share. I know the leaders would stay after class, and I know I could reach out to a pastor in my time of need, but somehow, this seems like too much to ask, especially if my worry is small.

There are book groups, prayer chains, and social opportunities galore, all intended to bring us closer to the heart of our faith. It's easy for me to get caught up in the moment when I'm with others, but I've found group activities leave me longing for the one-on-one relationship I imagine I could have with God.

What do you do when you can't sense the Spirit walking with you or feel lost and alone?

I heard about spiritual direction a few years back when a writer I followed worked to obtain her certification in the discipline. I didn't think twice about it because I didn't have a need at that time. Until recently, I'd never considered the benefits of working with a spiritual director. I assumed I should have a need before seeking help. What I didn't know is that the primary purpose of a spiritual director is not to "fix me" but to turn my focus to the One who can. They are often trained in various ways to support individuals seeking guidance on their journey with God.

I met Christy many years ago when she and her husband attended my gym. She was hard working and faithfully participated in the program, making it to the top five in her challenge group. She is a teacher, a beautiful writer, a hobby florist, and most recently, a student of Spiritual Direction. I wasn't surprised when I discovered she was spreading her wings this way. I've always known her to be quiet, thoughtful, and happy, even when she walked into the gym at 4:45 am! She appreciates natural beauty and is active in her local church.

I visited with her to learn why she was called to this course of study. She joined a contemplative community a few years back as she was looking to strengthen her prayer practices and benefitted from a guide of her own.

I asked about the role of a spiritual director and how she hoped to use her certification in the future. She said a spiritual director is different from a pastor or a counselor. They serve in a way that facilitates a relationship rather than working to solve a problem. She hopes to serve as a trusted companion for others looking for guidance as they deepen their spiritual practice and provide a safe space for those who may be at a crossroads. "I want to help people find a closer connection to God. That doesn't mean providing them with an answer, Spiritual direction always points you back to yourself, and sometimes that means not knowing the answer. My job is to serve as a companion; to pray with you, pray for you, and to reassure you that your hopes, dreams, and concerns are safe with me."

From a blog post at Faithlead.org, "Spiritual direction is charting God's presence in the story of your life. Lay and ordained people alike benefit from having a spiritual director, especially if you are discerning a big question in life such as "What does God want me to do now that I'm retired?" or "Am I called to the priesthood?" or "What does God want from me in my roles as mother, wife, and daughter?"— and everything in between. A spiritual director will also pray with and for you and sometimes give spiritual homework assignments to help you deepen your relationship with God."[6]

Spiritual direction differs from pastoral counseling, mentoring, and discipleship in that spiritual direction is not need-driven but focuses on the everyday experiences of the directee and the presence of God in those experiences.

A spiritual director can assist you in many ways:

- Clarifying your spiritual goals, values, and priorities.
- Identifying areas of growth and providing direction on how to achieve them.
- Providing accountability to your spiritual commitments and practices.
- Encouraging you to maintain a consistent spiritual routine.

- Helping you explore new ways to deepen your connection with God.
- Serving as a trusted mentor and guide on your spiritual path, offering support, insight, and encouragement as you navigate the complexities of your faith and personal growth.

I asked Christy what the most important thing was she'd like to share with my readers. She smiled, looked into my eyes, and said, "God loved you first."

Amen.

Wading In: Who do you turn to when you need direction?

Deep Dive: How is the Spirit working in your life?

Crowding Out for Prayer

1 minute:

- **Box Breath**

  Breathe in… 1…2…3…4

  Hold…1…2…3…4

  Breathe out…1…2…3…4

  Hold… 1…2…3…4

  Repeat twice

- **Angel Touch**

  11:11 or 4:44- whenever you see repeating numbers, stop whatever you're doing and chat with God for just a moment. I consider it a touch from a friend (kind of like a text):

  "Hello, my God. Thank you for letting me know you're thinking about me.

  I sense you near, and your presence brings me peace."

- **Prayer of Thanks**

  Oh God,

  Imagine my surprise when I turned over a beautiful shell, broken enough to reveal the bloom of spirals inside.

  The shell's purpose is complete, but the beauty in its transformation has brought me great joy. Thank you for reminding me that my life still has a great purpose.

  Help me find ways to change, grow, and bring joy to someone each day.

  Amen

- **Silence (single-word meditation)**

  Like Breath Prayer, inhale deeply and let your word escape on the exhale.

  Still

  Breathe

  Love

  Heal

- **God Bless**

  Like the good old days when you thought great things happened after you went to bed, Lift up the names of those who need an extra touch.

5 Minutes:

- **Breath Prayer**

  Based on techniques learned from *Breath as Prayer* by Jennifer Tucker[7]

  1. Breathe in slowly through your nose, filling your lungs. Exhale slowly- empty your lungs fully.

  2. Repeat until you achieve a slow, steady rhythm

3. Inhale the first part of your prayer, "The Lord is my Shepherd,"
4. Exhale: "I have all that I need."
5. Repeat

- **ACTS Prayer**

  Dear God,

  You are SO good.

  Forgive me for getting caught up in the busyness of my life.

  Thank you for this morning. Thank you for the joy in the ocean's calm and the shells' music.

  Thank you for the reminder we are beautiful in our brokenness.

  When we feel our purpose is complete, God, remind us we can begin anew and bring joy to others through those new beginnings.

  Help me to carry this joy into my day. Help me share it with those I encounter today. Help me to hold the peace I feel right now in my heart and to use it throughout the day. Remind me that my only duty is to love and forgive me when my temper flares, as you know it will. And help me, Lord, to live my life as a reflection of your love and sacrifice.

  I love you, and I'm so thankful you loved me first.

  Amen

- **Gratitude List**

  Jot down a predetermined number of things you're grateful for in a journal to wrap up the day. Three seems to be the magical number for many people: Today, I'm thankful for an unexpected rainstorm, honking geese chasing puppies on the path, and walkers who smiled as they passed!

10 Minutes:

- **Brisk Walk** Headphones off! Enjoy your surroundings.
- **Timed Prayer Journal** is a great way to connect. Set a timer and write all that's on your heart.
- **Gratitude Journal:** More than a list! Write about something that recently impacted your life. Use your senses!

30 Minutes:

- **Wander freely in Nature**

  Drive away from noise and distraction and walk for a while. Explore with your senses.

- **Morning Pages**

  There will be more about this in the next chapter, so this is just a bit of a tease! Morning pages first thing, clear the cobwebs and make my prayer life more fruitful.

- **Read Scripture**

  When I started reading scripture, I used prompts from a journal titled *Write the Word* from Cultivates What Matters[8]. I would work my way through, reading the assigned scripture and then copying the part that spoke to me in my journal. Now I'm reading the whole Holy Bible, in order with my church. I often highlight specific passages that stand out to me and write about one or two verses in my journal.

Chapter 2

Write it Down

Owner's Manual

My goal was not to write another diet book.

My goal is to share the processes I followed to achieve my goals and find joy in the journey. If you're like I am, you've undoubtedly tried many ways to shed a few pounds or tone up your body. The bookshelf in my kitchen is a testament to how many plans I've tried. The shelves are bowing with dozens of diet books that promise to make it easy.

I've followed plans over the years that have facilitated weight loss and increased strength, but I can't tell you they have succeeded. Why? Because I didn't enjoy the process enough to make the progress sustainable. Several of the programs recommended food tracking, but time and time again, I'd start and give up out of boredom.

I've been an off-and-on journaler throughout the years, but I didn't work to master keeping track of my food until I reached a breaking point in trying to overcome my auto-immune symptoms.

I developed psoriasis in my early twenties, and I have arthritis in my hands. I sensed my symptoms could be caused or controlled by the food I consumed, so I tracked them faithfully for many months. Somehow, trying to conquer more than the scale motivated me to record my meals regularly.

Through the process of writing it down, I learned what causes my auto-immune condition to flare. I also discovered that I achieve my weight loss goals quicker when I eat regular balanced meals comprised of unprocessed foods.

After I figured out my psoriasis triggers, I started to include additional details in my journals. I recorded my food, but also information about exercise, my period, and pre-menopausal symptoms. Suddenly, I realized the power of recording; I had history! I could make educated decisions and participate in medical appointments because I had knowledge about my body. I was no longer guessing when my doctors asked me a question because I had data.

And ladies, that is empowering. I have great doctors on my personal team, but no one knows me better than I do. I consider each completed journal another edition of Kim's Owners Manual. I can look back and see what foods allowed me to have incredible workouts or caused me to have disrupted sleep. I can see that the frequency of wine consumption causes night sweats, and regular walking directly correlates with more words on the page when I sit down to work. I have proof that the better I treat my body, the better it works for me.

Through the years, I've created a writing habit that includes personal journaling, including Morning Pages and Prayer, which I'll share more about later. I had separate journals for each type of writing, and it became cumbersome.

One of the most important things I've learned about myself is that I don't follow through if a habit isn't easy. I've also discovered I'm a more faithful contributor to one book than several. I return to my journal throughout the day more often than when I had a book for each part of my life. It is my constant companion, traveling in my purse or backpack, waiting as I create new recipes, and sleeping close by at night, just in case I have a fantastic breakthrough in my dreams!! The only thing I don't write in my journal is my grocery or to-do lists- those are created weekly on a sticky note on the front cover!

Through trial and error, I've discovered that I don't like spiral-bound notebooks and 8.5x11 journals because they don't fit in my bags. My journal has a soft leather cover and deliciously smooth lined pages that allow my pen to glide over magically, almost as if it's writing itself. I'm hoping you'll become a habitual journaler as well and that you'll write every day- not just on the days when your journal fits in your purse!

Wading In: Buy a journal and a really great pen. When will you write?

Deep Dive: Christen your new journal with a letter to your future self. What do you want to remember about the way you feel today?

♥

Why Write?

"It's a shame for a woman to grow old without ever seeing the strength and beauty of which her body is capable."

Socrates[1]

Take a second, break from reading and grab your owner's manual.

I'll wait here.

I'm waiting… still waiting. Are you coming back? What? You can't find it?

Ha, ha, funny, right? But not really.

Can you think of any one thing in your life that's more important than your body? Of course, your heart, mind, and soul, but I'm including all those when I say body.

Who taught you how to take care of the greatest gift you've ever been given? If your upbringing was like mine, no one really talked to you about the care and maintenance of your body. When you're young, your machine handles abuse, going miles on little fuel and even farther on no rest. You rebound from fender benders quickly, and your insurance claims are typically few and far between.

Over time, you start to notice a creak here or a twinge over there, and you're not quite sure what to do with it, so you head to the doctor. You might have an x-ray or a few tests, and likely, you'll leave with something to make you feel better. It might be a referral or an exercise, a lifestyle recommendation, or a prescription.

I'm all about modern medicine, and I'm grateful for those who have spent years learning to be doctors and therapists, but sometimes, I feel like our healthcare providers enable us to take the easy way out.

I know it's easy to take a pill, but isn't there just a little bit of you who would like to fix your problems without a prescription or a procedure? Journaling has given me the data I need to make the choices that are best for me.

Recently, after completing my yearly lab work, I had a back-and-forth with my primary doctor's nurse about the need for additional testing. One of the screening results seemed to be "a little high," and she advised me to conduct more tests. I have historical evidence in my journals and my medical chart showing my numbers are consistent at varying weights, enabling me to avoid unnecessary procedures.

Fortunately, I've reached a point in my life when I have a team of doctors willing to listen to me and entertain my observations about my body. It hasn't always been that way, but now that I have health information that covers an extended period through my journals, they are usually willing to work with me.

Unfortunately, I'm reaching an age where many of my peers are on medications. It seems that the expectation is to take a pill when things are out of whack, but that's not how I want to live my life or spend my money. The record of my behaviors and historical test results helps me remain in control of my health journey.

I eat a regular diet of protein, fat, carbs, and veggies, but I keep track so I know why I'm seeing changes or feeling stalled. Surprisingly, I experience the most significant progress when I eat regularly, three to four times a day. Less food is definitely not better for my weight loss goals.

As I mentioned, I write down more than just my food. Exercise, sleep, incontinence moments, and other changes are recorded. I included my monthly cycle when I still had one. Joint pain and headaches, hot flashes, and moodiness are in there too. I just started my first oral medication for psoriasis, and now I keep track of my skin condition so I can justify the cost and determine the benefit of a drug in my body.

Finally, I record my exercise. I like matching my activity up with the other things in my life. Some aches and pains are justified, like a sore hip after a five-mile beach walk. Others are something to pay attention to, like knee pain that won't go away no matter how much rest, ice, or ibuprofen I try.

I have an owner's manual created for my unique machine, and you should too.

I've worked with several women who had a journaling practice at one point or another in their lifetime, but many of them have given it up for various reasons. One friend told me she used to be an avid journaler, but the process had become cumbersome. She would spend hours re-reading and organizing at the expense of enjoying life. She burned her journals in the backyard fire-pit, releasing herself from the past they contained, and hasn't journaled since.

I polled a group of friends and learned there are many reasons they quit journaling:

Lack of Time: Busy schedules, family responsibilities, and work commitments often leave women feeling like they lack time for journaling.

Self-Criticism: Some women may become overly critical of their writing, feeling that their entries are not meaningful or well-written enough.

Privacy Concerns: Worries about someone else reading their journals.

Emotional Difficulty: Journaling often involves delving into emotions, which can be challenging or painful. Some women may quit because they find this emotional exploration uncomfortable.

I've slipped into downbeat rhythms, crying over pages and tearing portions out. But over time, I realized the good outweighed the bad, and I've faithfully been journaling for the last three years.

Below, I've listed a few reasons you might want to reconsider journaling again:

Emotional Outlet: Journaling provides a safe and private space to get it all out!

Creative Outlet: Journaling is a great way to explore creativity through writing, drawing, or praying.

Goal Setting and Tracking: Use journals to set goals, track progress, and celebrate!

Enhanced Communication: Journaling can improve communication skills. I often work through tough conversations on paper before meeting someone. I feel prepared and able to articulate my thoughts and feelings effectively.

Preserving Memories: Write to share your stories or remember them in the years to come!

Creativity and Inspiration: Journaling can help me when I'm stuck. Random free writing often produces an idea that helps me break through a block!

Ultimately, you have to do what works best for you. I know life flies by quickly, and I had difficulty keeping track of facts and losing grasp of great ideas too quickly for my liking. Consider if the potential benefits of writing outweigh your obstacles, and let me know if you decide to pick up your pen again!

Start creating your owner's manual.

Wading In: Include everyday occurrences like sleep or exercise

Deep Dive: Allow yourself to free-write at the end of your day. What did you learn about yourself today?

♥

Choose Your Audience

"Write down for the coming generation what the Lord has done, so that people not yet born will praise him."

Psalms 102:18

I am blessed to have had wonderful parents, step-parents, and grandparents, as well as many aunts and uncles in my life, each one adding their secret spice to the creation of me. I have memories of their laughs, the smell of their cologne, and their hugs.

My grandma passed away just a few years ago at the age of ninety-four, and although we spent a great deal of time together, I'm sad that I don't know more of her stories. It seems we were always busy cooking or catching up on current events- now that I have time to learn about the people who influenced her, she isn't here to share the details.

My mom has shared beautiful memories and photos from her childhood, and my stepmother recently sent me a book of pictures and historical information so I can begin to piece together a little more of my family tree. Still, I find myself longing for the stories…

I just became a grandma! My youngest son and his wife had a boy in August and my oldest son and his wife are expecting a boy in May. There is nothing better than those moments when I get to bury my nose in the little rolls on his neck and breathe in the baby sweetness. I dream about rolling around on the floor with them, playing peekaboo, and reading the treasured books hidden for years in anticipation of another child in my lap.

It dawned on me that I had hundreds of moments with my sons, and as cherished as those are, I didn't spend much time telling the boys my stories. They were learning, busy exploring, and suddenly, grown and gone. Family get-togethers often leak an embarrassing tale or two, but they don't know all of the moments or all of the people who made me who I am today, and quite honestly, they don't have time now to listen to my recollections. But someday, their lives will slow down, and they will sit and wonder where they come from and who shaped their lives.

The morning after I found out about Baby M, I started writing to him. I didn't know his gender or his due date. I didn't care… I lovingly wrote to my future grandchild about what was happening in my world and that of his parents. I barely touched on current events because those things can be found simply by entering a date into a search engine. I wrote because I want future generations of my family to know who I am and where I come from. I want them to have a treasure to turn to someday when I'm gone. I started another journal when I found out about Baby C and I will continue with each grandchildren to come.

There isn't a structure to my writing, just occasional entries to share a story, often about something his daddy did that will make him laugh. Sometimes, it's about an incredible place he should visit when he's older or a movie he should watch. As I continue to write, I'll include books I love, songs he should know, and recipes for the cookies he will help me make.

I end each entry with a prayer.

I want my grandchildren to know how faithful God has been to me and to learn that they can trust Him to listen to their sorrows and celebrate their joys. I want them to know I trust God to watch over them when I'm not near, and even though life will bring them sadness, they can count on the never-ending love of One greater than their sorrow.

I met a lovely woman recently. She has a beautiful story about the power of written prayers.

Lisa is a faithful Christian- one of those people who goes beyond saying she'll pray for me and actually does it right there in the room or over the phone so I can listen (I want to be like her in this way, but that's a work in progress too).

She has been battling health issues for decades, not knowing the cause and, therefore, not knowing the cure or even how to reduce the symptoms. She lost her mother too early, but in her passing, my friend discovered journals that prayerfully included requests in her name. The power of a mother's love and her faith in Jesus are available long after the words can be spoken out loud. My friend has a forever piece of her mother's faith anytime she feels overwhelmed and alone.

I want to offer that to my family. I can't be with them every time I include them in my prayers, but through these special journals, I hope to give my present and future family hope, comfort, and the realization that they are forever in my heart. I believe in His faithfulness, entrusting their care to God, knowing he will hold them long after I'm gone.

Wading In: Write a story about your childhood.

Deep Dive: Change your audience. Share a story from your life with someone you love.

♥

Morning Pages

My brain works best at 5:00 am. It also functions sufficiently later in the day, but somehow, in the still warm-from-bed fog of the morning, I write freely, capturing most of the words I find worthy of sharing before the sun rises. I'd like to tell you it's because I'm an avid dreamer, and my creative side likes the dark of the night, but I think it's more logical to credit early mornings at the gym. I learned a lot about myself in the wee hours while driving to work. Allowing myself to think in silence first thing each day has been one of the greatest gifts of my life.

I traveled solo to California in March 2021 to attend a writing retreat at The Oaks with two of my favorite authors, Bob Goff and Kimberly Stuart, and twenty other creatives. It wasn't my inaugural trip alone, but it was the first one when I wasn't meeting a friend on the other side of the country.

It was also the first time I dreamed of becoming a writer.

I arrived, administered my first-ever COVID test (thankfully passed), and checked in for the three-day adventure. I chose to room alone because I like to write at 5:00 am, which is 3:00 in California! And also because I'm pretty sure I snore!

On the bed in my room, there was a water bottle, a journal, a mini beach ball, and a copy of *The Artist's Way* by Julia Cameron[2]. I set my welcome package aside and floated through the weekend, talking to other writers, eating wonderful food, petting horses, and writing in the silence of nature. It was heaven!

I opened her book for the first time on the plane ride home. It was easy to settle into, and I skipped the prompts for more information. I loved the randomness of her suggestions, "*write three pages longhand, stream-of-consciousness morning writing*," just for the sake of writing!

In all honesty, I have to admit it was hard to take off my editor hat. I wanted to write something beautiful and grammatically correct every morning, but that wasn't the point. At first, I struggled to find something to fill the pages because I had never given myself permission to write for the heck of it. Sometimes, I feel a little crazy about the way ideas bounce back and forth on the page, but the meandering of my mind usually comes to complete focus by the time I sign off. I end every entry with a kiss and a hug (xo)- an attempt to love myself the way I should.

I've found great freedom in writing the way she described and have made morning pages a faithful part of my routine. Cameron suggests that the pages shouldn't be reread or shared, but I've discovered over time that my creativity spills out on the pages and can help me work through areas where I might be stuck in my public writing.

She also claims, "*When we open ourselves to exploring our creativity, we open ourselves to God: good orderly direction.*[3]" I believe she's right. I find that through writing, whether it's this book, written for you, or my journals, written for me, I've been able to come closer to God. I find myself wondering if the message I'm sharing does justice to the gifts He's offered me. I've opened my heart through the process to understand that my strengths were not simply meant for self-preservation; they were also gifted to help others.

Without the freedom learned through daily scribbling, I wouldn't have reached the clarity to put these words on the page.

There have been additional advantages as well. Through the regular clearing of the cobwebs each morning, I've discovered I have better focus as I start my day. I used to struggle to settle my mind, but by releasing my frustrations, joys, and ideas fully onto the page, I can calm my brain and emotions to learn or feel other things. There are mornings when my mind is quiet after Morning Pages- on those days, I read scripture. There are days when an idea is crystal clear after writing- on those days, I blog or write a chapter. There are also times when a new idea surfaces, and on those days, I like to walk, giving myself more time to work through the concept. I feel like whatever I choose to do is more on point.

As we begin our journey together, I'd challenge you to start each morning by purging your brain of everything that comes into it for the first thirty minutes of your day. I know you think you don't have time, but try. Set the alarm thirty to sixty minutes earlier than necessary, settle into a quiet space with a cup of coffee or tea, and write everything that pops into your head.

Cameron says to write three full pages, but in my world, there are no rules- except that you hold the time sacred. No disruptions. Create a time in the day that doesn't have anyone else's agenda attached to it. Do it before you open your phone. Do it before you check the weather. Do it when the thoughts in your mind are yours and only yours. You might be amazed at what flows onto the page.

Wading In: Start your day with morning pages.
Draw, doodle, make lists, anything works!

Deep Dive: Set a thirty-minute timer, and don't stop writing!
How much did you have to say?

♥

Write Now

Have you ever noticed you remember you need toilet paper when you're sitting in church? Or an amazing recipe idea reveals itself to you while waiting in the doctor's office in a paper gown with your bag on the chair, under a pile of clothes??

I am an avid note taker. Before cell phones, I had a notebook in each room, my bag, and the car. I would think of something and write it down. It's not a to-do list, but a don't-forget list. Truth be told, I had so many notebooks and lists I rarely had the one I needed at the time. I've learned what works best for me is one journal that can be used for any thought- morning writing, recipes, prayers, and blog ideas fill the pages.

I have a friend who uses two journals: one for creative writing and another for data entry (her owner's manual). I recently learned while listening to a podcast that another Iowa-based writer uses nine different journals regularly! She prefers to keep her subjects separate.

The most important thing is to create a practice that works for you.

Sometimes, having a journal with you is impractical, like at the gym or on a walk. But, because my phone is with me wherever I go, I have a mini-computer at my disposal 24 hours a day. I've consolidated my random thoughts and anything else I don't want to forget on the notes app on my phone.

I've written speeches, created blog posts, and outlined entire chapters as I move through my day, piece by piece, when a thought catches me. Sometimes, I type it in. Other times, I dictate. "Writing" doesn't have to be accomplished in complete silence at a desk with a keyboard. The best ideas can show up in the middle of a busy grocery store, as you're speeding down the highway, or strolling around a lake on a morning walk.

In a perfect world, we'd all have two hours of uninterrupted "free time" to write, correspond, and record our deepest thoughts and wildest dreams, but perfect worlds don't exist. You can either make do with using what you have available or lose your brilliant ideas and treasured thoughts to the wind.

Notes App: I love this feature on my cell phone; it has quickly become my most used app. The best thing is my notes transfer seamlessly to my laptop for easy editing and pasting into my manuscript. I'm unfamiliar with other brands, but a quick Google search indicates most smartphone brands have similar apps. There are paid apps as well, but I'm guessing the promised accuracy would take out the fun of trying to figure out what you really said when the app heard you say Chewbacca or Lalalala!

Recorder: I purchased a basic recorder. It doesn't have all the bells and whistles, but it works for me because it's compact and easy to operate. I've written large sections of this book while walking and have been able to participate fully in interviews because I didn't have to take notes. Most smartphones also have built-in recording capabilities, but I like that I can plug my recorder into my computer, and it will happily transcribe my notes into my manuscript!

Journal: A paper journal is still my favorite way to work through my thoughts and ideas. There's nothing better than the feel of a book in my hand. Soft and flexible with smooth pages, begging to be written on. I love them so much I have a delegated shelf in my bookcase for the blank ones. I used to have separate journals for everything. Recipes in one, prayers in another, and workout routines in yet a third. Now that I'm writing everything in one journal, I have an efficient reflection of my life for a small window of time. It's easy to flip through to find specific information or a memory.

Who knows, maybe someday, when I'm long gone, my journals will be published and offered in the humor, self-help, spiritual, cooking, exercise, and random thoughts section of a bookstore near you!

I recently ordered a pen with a soft light on the end to capture those late-night, dream-inspired revelations without getting up or opening my phone app. I'm so excited! I imagine late-night moments of brilliant writing as I record my dreams! *Update: It's terrible! Imagine trying to capture your profound sleep revelations with a spotlight in your way. I don't think I saw clearly for days after using it!*

Sticky Notes: Has there ever been a better invention? I love sticky notes! I carry them with me wherever I go for quick thoughts, a simple thank you to a server, or an addition to a journal post that I want to be recorded in the correct historical time. My recipe entries often have stickies that detail delicious variations or timing changes.

Wading In: Create a backup plan for your writing.

Deep Dive: Compile your "on-the-fly" notes into your journal. Did they provide clarity to an earlier question?

♥

Do It "Write"

I'm what I like to call a multi-dimensional learner. I read for knowledge, watch for understanding, and get my hands dirty for mastery. Listening is my weakest link (just ask my parents!).

I find it frustrating to read a book filled with great ideas only to be left feeling empty at the end because I don't know if I'm doing it "right."

You'll discover through this book that I don't believe in right and wrong, and I rarely play in the land of black and white. I've learned to live quite happily in the world of gray possibilities! Trial and error reign supreme in this place, and slowly, my need for perfection is fading away.

But just in case you haven't arrived here, I thought I'd share a day in the life of my journal. Enjoy, and remember, no judgment!

Thursday, April 13~ woke late. Alarm was set for five to write, but I guess I needed more sleep! The sun was just starting to streak the sky with pink when I crawled out of bed. It's good to be home, though I think the bed at the condo in Florida was better than this one. My back aches and I don't feel as rested. Should be a good day to write- Jeff's going golfing and the housework is done. What a great party Saturday- so fun to see Madi & Sam's friends and to finally find out Baby M is a boy! I wish he were here now, but I remember how I needed ALL nine months to prepare.

Lots of ideas are running through my head for new books- it would be nice if my brain could wrap itself around reflections long enough for me to get it sent off to TJ. Next week should be the week... I'm going to silence my socials, print the chapters and read- I hope I like it ;)

I need to get better with my IG posts. It seems like I have to choose between manuscript words and social words. Maybe it's that I get sucked in when I go on to post. I like so much of it, but hate so much at the same time... but no matter how I feel about social media, I know it has power over me and my schedule. I hope the baby doesn't get to play with the phone. I saw an interview yesterday (on IG!!) about neural targeting- how created technology inhibits free spontaneous creative play and gets them hooked as early as the age of one!

Zach and Jenny have both quit their socials... both seem happy with the decision. I know how important they are to promoting the book- maybe I can automate my posts more once the manuscript has moved into editing.

I had a great convo with Lisa yesterday. Trying to figure out some accountability steps so I can submit before leaving for the conference. I like the idea of letting someone in my target audience read before I submit... but honestly, I don't want to read anyone's comments and be thrown into a phase of justification.

Stinks to know myself so well. It was easier when I was young and sure everything I did was right! Ha!

My back is aching- I need to get back outside. It was so much easier to walk on the beach. Rainy and cold again today- sun's supposed to come out later- maybe a walk before lunch.

Caught up on my Bible reading- the old testament pace is hard to keep up with- but once I start reading, it sucks me in... I can NOT believe the things that happened. So much fighting. Hard to switch gears from the battles in 1 & 2 Samuel to the love of John. Note to self: DON'T FALL BEHIND!!

For now... xoxo

Breakfast- 2 eggs, sourdough, sauteed spinach, cherry tomatoes, grapes and pineapple, 2 coffee

Walk full circle @ Ada

Right hip still aching-

Allergies are terrible - perfect time to come back to Iowa- cold AND pollen.

Psoriasis seems to be flaring too- I wonder if I should switch meds?

1:11 Heavenly Father, You are so good! Thank you for the warmth of the sun and the push to get outside. I've felt stuck since I got home... remind me of the words I promised myself when I was still at the beach! My health is important no matter where I am- help me to remain faithful to my goals. Please watch over Kat's mom as she travels to Florida- I'm not sure when she flies, but keep her safe and give her warmth and beautiful weather while she's there. Please watch over those closest to my heart- help them find joy in this day.

I love you, and I'm so thankful you love me. Amen.

Lunch- flat bun, turkey, swiss, garlic aioli, spinach, carrots, avocado mash, half orange- too full

New bread recipe- added roasted garlic in tucks at 2 and 4 hours... smells good. I hope it tastes good.

Dinner- cooked chicken wild rice soup- went to see Sam and Madi's new house, so ate dinner with them instead. They are working hard to save money, so we all decided we could eat what they planned! We don't have to go out, even if we are celebrating! We had roast, potatoes, and carrots when we got back to Ames. Glass of wine when I got home. I'm afraid of a long day tomorrow helping pack and move.

NEED to remember to call carpet cleaner and internet people- UGH! Keep forgetting!

Go As A River... getting good! Will have to pass to the girls when I'm done.

New shrub idea- simple syrup with monk fruit, cranberries and orange peel, red wine vinegar. It would be good w/ the sparkling orange water I found in the cupboard!

Blessings:

1. New House for Sam and Madi (new opportunity for us w/ condo)

2. Growing BABY! I saw ALL of the sonogram pics tonight
3. My walk... gorgeous roots of the big tree in the west pond. Silence and Sunshine

♥

Crowding Out to Write

1 minute:

- **Capture your dream!** Write down the bright, shiny details as soon as you wake. They are enough to spark your memory later in the day.
- **Leave yourself a note.** Record a reminder, a memorable quote, or a question you need to remember.

5- 10 Minutes:

- **Write while on hold.** Think about the times you sit and wait on hold, often for five minutes or more. I set a timer for 5 minutes and typed at will, not about anything, and achieved 201 words within the five minutes (and I'm a terrible typer!) The popular November writing challenge, *NaNoWriMo* (National Novel Writing Month)[4], began in 1999 as a daunting but straightforward challenge: to write 50,000 words of a novel in thirty days! This can be accomplished by writing 1667 words/ day for 30 days. Just think, you could write your masterpiece minutes at a time!
- **Talk on hold.** Just because I thought it would be fun, I set a five-minute timer and used Google Voice to write- I achieved 624 words in five minutes this way!
- **Train time.** Write in your journal while waiting on the train or in the pick-up line at school.

30 Minutes:

- **Morning Pages**. Start your day off right!

- **Gratitude Journal.** Skip scrolling or TV time. Close the night by writing about at least three things that made you happy throughout the day.

♥

Chapter 3

Reflections

Who Are You?

Millions of women pray for weight loss. Most have no idea about the emotional changes that come with physical change. They just want to feel pretty, skinny, sexy… loved.

They diet and exercise, and soon they fit into smaller clothes, then sexier clothes. People pay attention to them. Suddenly, they are no longer invisible.

Sadly, most women aren't prepared for the changes in their relationships, and they have no way to clear their memories of the hurtful things they've felt or heard.

It's incredible what people say with their eyes when you're overweight and then with their mouths when you get skinny. It's even more incredible what you can't forget.

Hundreds of new members walked through my door each year when I ran my gym. Many of those were challengers. If you participated in our nine-week program, you would take before and after photos to be eligible to win the grand prize. 99% of the time, I took the photos, and even though I had endured my own pictures on more than a couple of occasions, I still felt anxious for the person in front of my lens.

I would do my best to make them feel comfortable:

"Hi, I'm Kim! This will go quickly, I promise! Stand like this *click*. Turn like this *click*. Now, like this *click*. Good! You're done!"

Some challengers joked with me, some hinted at a smile with teary eyes, and others wouldn't look at the lens; they fixed their gaze on a phantom spot on the wall. Almost all of them would share how awful they thought they looked or mused about how disappointed they were about letting themselves go. I can't recall a single time when someone said: "Thanks, I can't wait to see these."

Many women refused to take pictures. They weren't in it for the competition. They were simply looking for better health. I understood but also encouraged them to take photos and measurements for themselves simply because you can't look in the mirror and take an accurate snapshot of what you look like at a specific moment in time.

Competition or not, you deserve to see your accomplishments after a period of hard work.

When the last challenger had been photographed, I would take the memory card out of the camera and store it away, waiting until the last week of the challenge to download and crop. I'm still amazed at the changes that occur when someone chooses good food, regular movement, sleep, and friendship.

We would record markers such as weight and body fat during initial testing and chart specific measurements. We'd also test performance on push-ups, sit-ups, and a mile walk/run. Finally, I handed out a questionnaire that asked for basic information and guided clients to reflect on several questions, including the following:

- What do you do for fun?
- What kind of music do you like?
- What are your favorite foods and drinks?
- What are three things you love about yourself?
- What are three things you'd like to change?
- What are your goals for the next several weeks?

In 90% of the questionnaires, one line was always left blank. Can you guess which one?

Based on my experience, it was the same one I left blank on my first challenge and the same one you didn't answer:

What are three things you love about yourself?

This lack of self-love makes it hard for people to make lasting changes. We're so hesitant to look in the mirror and appreciate the good that's there. We dream of long, lean bodies with defined muscles and supple, blemish-free skin with no signs of under-eye circles, smile lines, or droopy... well, droopy anything.

We live in a social world where we're exposed more than ever to opinions, breaking news, and unverified promises made by exercise and diet influencers. It's easy to feel caught in the middle when you try to embark on a new health and wellness journey. One post makes us feel ugly and ashamed, a gimmick diet post makes us feel deceived, and yet another might make us secretly repulsed by unhealthy attitudes.

You may have received "the talk" from your doctor about the fact that your test scores are borderline or that a life of prescription drugs is inevitable. You receive enough guidance to know you have to lose weight but not enough information to know how. You have tried every diet, workout, and supplement you can get your hands on. You lose weight only to gain it back again because you are too busy to keep up with the rigor of fad diets, and your middle-aged body can't recover from ninety-minute cardio sessions the way it used to! Add to the mix that your hormones are all over the place! You just want to be active and healthy, to feel strong and confident, and to look in the mirror and feel beautiful.

As a coach, I interacted with women of all ages with varying goals. Some wanted to lose weight, some wanted to gain muscle, and others hoped to get off meds. I watched some people change for the better in their health. Muscle definition, better athletic form, brighter eyes, and a confident stride were often the telltale signs that showed up first.

Other members would get frustrated when they focused too much on the scale. They would practice deprivation or over-exercising to achieve weight loss results faster than the others. Their spirit often suffered because their methods were lonely and unsustainable. Over time, weight would creep back up, or their body would break down. Some women would give up, citing age and hormones or lack of time and money. I heard what their mouths said when they quit but often observed something entirely different. It's hard to want more changes than your body will offer. It's hard to not be perfect.

Wading In: Who Are You?

Deep Dive: Answer the following questions in your journal:

- What is your name?
- Where do you work?
- Who are your people? Names and ages, please!
- Do you have pets?
- When is your birthday?
- What is your favorite color?
- What do you do for fun?
- What kind of music do you like?
- What are your favorite foods and drinks?
- What are three things you love about yourself?
- What are three things you'd like to change?
- What are your goals for the next several weeks?

♥

Look In the Mirror

"...one of the qualities that makes human beings so unique out of all other living species is our capacity to reject being ourselves. To hide our identity. To put on a mask and pretend to be something we're not."

Happy Advent by Scott Erickson[1]

Body Positivity is a growing movement today, as it should be. Each human is a gift, their bodies beautiful and unique. I would be surprised if any other creature gazes at its reflection, thinks, "I'm not worthy," and goes out of its way to change.

But somewhere in the celebration of *everybody*, there has to be a discussion about responsibility. Body positivity should be a celebration of what our bodies are capable of, not an entitlement to push our bodies to unrealistic limits. Our basic skeletal frame is not meant to bear the burden of excessive weight. Our hearts were not created to sit at rest, and our brains were not designed to stare at screens for hours at a time.

We have a responsibility to take care of the body we've been given. If we came with an owner's manual, it would undoubtedly provide guidance on the right fuel, safe use, and regular check-up schedule.

Hopefully, you've begun creating such a manual, and I will lead you using the assumption that you want to make changes to improve your health.

Nothing in the following pages is meant to diminish the beautiful differences we possess, but it will lean towards best practices of eating whole food, daily movement, quality rest, cultivating relationships, mental growth, and spiritual engagement.

It's easy to lose weight. I know because I've done it at least one hundred times! The trick comes in finding a way to settle into a healthy, happy, and sustainable place. Our natural bodies are incredible machines; most of us are born with the ability to overcome health issues with time, care, and occasional medicine.

It's important to reflect on what's good in us and to use it as the foundation to build the rest, so that's where we'll begin. And because I know you have to learn to walk before you run, I used the word "like" in this first chapter, but my goal is for you to be able to love yourself long before you reach your goal.

The point of the following exercise is to capture your best self, the way you are today. I want you to look for the woman you catch in the mirror on a good day and think, "Hmm, I'm not so bad!" You'll never be able to scroll back in your memories to examine yourself closely without the automatic photo-enhancing quality of your brain altering your reality. You may create a memory linked to emotion, but it will lose the details of your beautiful eyes, strong shoulders, and pretty toes.

Fix your hair the way you like. Approach the camera awake and fresh-faced, or add some mascara and a little lipstick if that's what you do. Select clothing that makes you feel beautiful and confident. If you can't yet begin to think about yourself that way, choose something that makes you feel comfortable.

Take a picture or have someone who loves you do it for you. Then, set your camera to the side and look at yourself. *Really* look. Start at the top of your head and work your way down… what do you see? For everything you'd like to change, I'd encourage you to find something you like. Here's my list:

LIKE	LIKE TO CHANGE
I like the color of my hair	I'd like to wear my hair shorter
I love my eyes- they make me Me!	I wish I had just one chin
I like my smile	I wish my arms were more toned
I have broad shoulders	I wish my chest was smaller
I have good posture	I would like to get rid of my pooch
I have good calf muscles	I wish my rear was smaller
I have pretty toes	

Okay! Your turn. Seriously, don't skip this part. No matter how bad you feel about yourself or how disappointed you may be in your current state of being, there are several good things! Get out your Owner's Manual and reflect on these as you make your lists. Look at yourself as you would a friend:

LIKE	LIKE TO CHANGE

Now, you've looked at yourself, so sit down and think about the following questions:

1. What do you like about yourself (not physical, for example, "I am a nice person" or "I am a good mom")?

   ____

2. Is there anything from your past you would like to escape or forget?

    ____

3. What would you change in your life? (Health? Career? Relationships? Activities?)

    ____

4. How will your life suffer if you don't change?

    ____

5. How will your life be better if you succeed?

    ____

6. What is the one thing you're unwilling to give up to realize your goal?

    ____

You've looked in the mirror, and you identified not only your gifts but also your opportunities. Several years ago, when I managed a restaurant, we'd gather at the end of every shift to discuss "wells and betters." What went well? What could have gone better? Consider your self-evaluation the same way. How does my body perform well? What do I like about myself? What could be better? What are potential roadblocks, and what are the rewards?

It doesn't get any harder than that.

If you completed the list, well done!

If not, think about the questions for a while

and return to this exercise.

You'll be glad you did.

Skip the Scale

Several of you might be confused about why we didn't step on a scale. Others might wonder why I didn't ask you to squeeze into a sports bra and compression shorts to take measurements.

I've become a big believer in positive reinforcements and non-scale victories.

I know my body is different every single day of my life. I know that I eat different foods and consume varying amounts of water. I know that salt and caffeine and lack of sleep or inflammation can nudge the scale one way or the other from day to day. I also know how hard it is to give up everything you like to eat in the name of a new number and not have it happen.

Anticipation about a weigh-in after a stellar week of eating often ends in disappointment if the stars aren't aligned just so. We give the scale an awful amount of power for something that doesn't have a brain. Its entire purpose is to measure mass. It doesn't differentiate between muscle, water, or fat. Weight is simply a number, so I no longer use it as a measuring stick for success.

You can weigh yourself if you wish, but please don't get on that darn thing every day. Create a habit of weighing on the same day of the week (or month), at the same time of day, with the same clothes (or lack of clothes), and give yourself grace for working on your health even if the dial doesn't move as much as you'd like. I step on the scale on the first day of every month just to keep my data-based brain happy.

I've had clients make remarkable changes. They became stronger and healthier, and some were even able to "describe" or omit medications from their daily routine.

****Please note: you should never discontinue a medication without discussing it with your physician. Several common medications should be reduced slowly under their careful watch, and others can be eliminated after appropriate tests have been performed.**

Other clients were so fixated on a number that they would throw their hands up, waving the white flag of surrender. They would return to their old habits because "nothing works anyway."

The part of this that makes me sad is that they were changing. I could see it in the number of reps before failure, with increased time in a plank, with the bagginess of their workout shirt- but they didn't give themselves time and didn't have the unedited Day One photo stored in their memory.

When I was twenty, I worked full-time. I didn't have time to exercise, and I often ate fast food during breaks at work. I remember stepping on the scale the day Mom and I shopped for a wedding dress. I hadn't exercised regularly in a few years but was happy with my weight and size. Fast forward twenty-five years. I exercised four to five days a week and ate unprocessed, whole foods ninety percent of the time. I weighed thirty pounds more than I did in my twenties and wore a smaller size.

The point of this is to illustrate the scale doesn't tell you the whole story. I could be happy at age forty-five about the way I looked and the way my body performed, or I could have beat myself up if the number on the scale was higher than in the past.

The way you feel about yourself makes all the difference in your success. Since I abandoned daily weigh-ins and chose to focus on non-scale victories (NSV), my body is changing. Somehow, choosing happiness and gratitude is impacting my weight.

No, I don't believe I can will away weight with a smile and a song in my heart, but choosing movement, food, and activities that bring me joy makes me want to return to them again and again. Habits are falling into place because I'm finally enjoying the process rather than focusing on my heart rate, number of steps, or calories consumed.

One of the most rewarding parts of my job was meeting people I wouldn't normally come in contact with. Many would join because a friend had shared their success, and they would show up ready to make some changes! They would share their stories and frustrations throughout the challenge and trust me to help them.

Nothing was better than seeing the scowls and tears that accompanied my new friends on the first day turn into smiles and sass by day thirty and into confidence and pride by day sixty when I took their "after photos."

Early in my career, shortly after opening the gym, a lovely, quiet woman and her daughter signed up for the challenge. They worked out together, and I'd often catch the athletic teen encouraging her mom on the bag, a smile here or an eye roll there. I'm unsure who wanted to sign up and who came along for moral support, but they worked together like best friends.

As was the case with many interrelated pairs, one liked to work out, and the other liked to cook. Mom was formerly a teacher who chose to stay home and raise her children. She often talked about her loving husband and great kids, and why she wanted to become more fit. She was a planner, which worked out great for her daughter, who benefitted from having a workout partner who also cooked for the family. Amy was a faithful journaler and recorded more than her meals, creating a historical account of her nine-week challenge.

I had the privilege to be one of her coaches, so I was privy to the transformation that occurred throughout her challenge. She went from setting weight goals to experiencing real-life body changes, and it was so much fun to watch! The following is from a food journal entry I saved because it inspired me so much; Some may have thought "only nine pounds", but as she wrote this, she was starting to see a difference in her body.

"I checked my weight today, and I was at XXX, which is a total of 9 lost so far. I wore my dress slacks to church on Sunday and decided I needed to go down a size because I had to pull them up constantly. So I am down one size in my jeans and my dress slacks woo hoo! As much as I would love to see that "unimportant number" on the scale go down faster for as much work as I think I am putting into this, I am definitely seeing a difference in my body size, and I am very happy with that."

Later entries would mention the realization that health benefits were surfacing and excitement about seeing her before photos. She knew she was changing even if the number on the scale wasn't dropping as much as she hoped. She worked hard to listen to my warnings to keep fueling the fire; she ate when she was hungry, even on the days the scale didn't honor her hard work with a drop.

She had incredible results and surpassed all her goals except for one. I don't have to tell you which one; she missed her weight-loss goal by less than five pounds, but her results confirmed what I already knew- the scale is nothing but a tool to measure mass. It doesn't measure strength, health, mood, or pant size!

She walked into the challenge party looking like a completely different woman. She was beautiful the day I met her, but the woman who showed up that night was striking, confident, and satisfied. She was a winner before I called her name, and she solidified the value of non-scale victories for me for the first time as a coach.

Our bodies are incredible machines! They'll change in ways you never dreamed of in a very short time if you give them good food, daily movement, and a positive outlook. Many things occur between the milestone moments of the before and after pictures:

- You notice your endurance improves, allowing you to exercise longer between breaks.
- You stand taller as your posture improves- suddenly, you don't feel like hiding- you like how your muscles feel strong, carrying you gracefully.
- You have more energy and bounce into class instead of dragging.
- You feel stronger- that 50# bag of dog food is suddenly no big deal!
- You catch your reflection in a store window and smile.
- You learn to anticipate your body's response to movement (hunger, soreness) and plan appropriately.
- You get "woozy" during class. I always recommend keeping your physician in the loop; many will discover their blood pressure or sugar response improves in a few short weeks (CHEERS to fewer meds!).
- You miraculously find time to cook. "I'm not going to waste a good workout with take-out."
- You sleep better.
- Your flexibility improves- you can paint your toenails for the first time in years!
- You look forward to workouts.

The best day of the challenge was always day sixty-one. With the final photo shoot complete, I would schedule the day to match and crop photos. I'd sit alone at the old desktop in the basement, with Kleenex in hand- a private moment for the photographer to witness all of the good that can be captured with the click of a button.

Of course, I could see what they lost… less hips and belly, smaller faces and fannies, but that's not really what mattered to me. It was the gain I was looking for. You know, the additions to the picture- the smile that replaced a frown or the new gleam in their eyes. The one that told me they were beginning to love themselves again but hadn't yet realized it.

Look in the mirror, take the picture, and pay attention to how your life changes. You'll be glad you did.

Wading In: Think about a non-scale victory.
What is something wonderful you dare to hope for?

Deep Dive: Expand on your answer above.
Why do you want to change?

The Friend

Each of us has that one friend who keeps you on your toes. You know the one. She looks fit without effort, has a beautiful smile, always looks put together, and is gracious and loving to everyone she meets. You feel flattered when she asks you to meet her for lunch, and you are inspired to look your best with her. She is perfect in every way, and you just can't get over how great her life is. Yet, if you could read her mind, you'd discover she's just like you, and there is a list of things she doesn't like about herself.

When I was younger, I used to say things like "I feel fat" or "I look gross," never thinking about how my negative self-talk hurt me, deep down where only my heart remembers. Those words affected me long-term as much as any spoken by another person. The more you put yourself down, the more you believe it and act it out.

Later on, when I was coaching, I witnessed the damage negative self-talk had on others. Trim, athletic members would be talking amongst themselves, grumbling about how a weekend of over-indulgence made them bloated. "I can't believe how fat I look" slipped out more times than I would have hoped into the earspace of an unsuspecting challenger. I could see the doubt creep into their expression as if to say, "What does she think about me?"

Until you learn to love yourself enough to eliminate the bashing, learn to silence it. I guarantee that someone in your circle of friends considers you their inspiration. Maybe they weigh more than you. Maybe they're struggling to find life balance. Maybe, just maybe, they'd give just about anything to live the life you have. When you put yourself down in front of them, imagine how they think you look at them.

Let's discuss something else while I'm on a roll: There is One who thinks you're perfect. He loves you like no one else ever could. He sees your potential, beauty, and goodness, and it breaks his heart that you can't see it in yourself.

After my first challenge, I thought "fit was it" (and it was, I suppose, for as long as it lasted). This time, I'm attempting to change how I view myself, noting the progress instead of focusing on the areas that still need work. I started listening to my husband, sons, and friends, who were all cheering me on. Initially, it was hard to change how I viewed myself, but over time, it's become easier to believe I'm beautiful just as I am.

A big part of looking the way you want is believing that you can make changes and setting yourself up for success. This starts with making your health and happiness a priority, and for some reason, it's something many women have a hard time accomplishing. If you're like I am, every time you get in a groove, the forces of the universe conspire to throw you off track. I'd read about women who made appointments with themselves, but I didn't do it myself until recently.

Figure out what works for you and stick to it whether you're tired, out of town, or in the middle of a big project at work. Give yourself enough room to modify your plan, but don't walk away. Learn to put yourself first regarding your health, and you'll stop the yo-yo you've been riding on.

It's vital to **Plan your Week**. Sit down at some point every weekend and look at the week ahead. You need to know when you have time to cook and workout and when social obligations might force you to alter your routine. If you still have kids at home, it's critical to include the whole family in the process. It's much easier to plan a different workout time when you know in advance. If you don't plan, you won't go.

Another vital piece of the pie is to **Simplify your Routines**. Pack a bag for the gym. Put your keys in the same place every night. Make several lunches at a time. Freeze baggies of fruit for your morning smoothie. Learn to "make up your face" with five products (seriously- moisturizer, mineral foundation, blush, mascara, and lipstick. Simple and beautiful.). Double a dinner recipe- cool half and freeze it for a busier night. Work hard to follow these routines until they become a habit.

Finally, **Surround Yourself with Support!** There's nothing worse than sitting in someone's driveway at 5 am on a cold, rainy day unless, of course, you're the one inside the house who forgot to set an alarm, rushing around in the dark trying to find your sports bra; I doubt your friendship will end over a random snooze button, but it's not a good way to start the day. Fortunately, if I know someone is waiting for me, I will wake up (often before the alarm).

Whether you carpool or drive separately, find a buddy as you begin your journey, Hold one another accountable, and share the load by swapping healthy meals, making after-workout snacks, or planning date nights together. It's easier to find the good stuff when sharing the load with a friend.

If you don't have an accountability partner or someone cheering you on at home, I strongly encourage you to sign up for at least one group fitness class each week or work with a personal trainer occasionally. Positive feedback and accountability are crucial for continued motivation in the gym, and it just feels good to have someone in your corner!

Wading In: How can you be "that friend"?
List ways you can support others who are on your journey.

Deep Dive: How could you use help from a friend?

♥

This is Me

In my opinion, nothing is more compelling than a confident woman. I can't help but admire someone who knows who she is, how she wants to look, and what she believes. I love the way she walks into a room and commands attention without saying a word.

I used to believe this woman must have a bursting bank account, a personal stylist, and a life coach. As I've paid closer attention, I've come to realize, more often than not, she has simply embraced *who* she is.

I want to be that woman.

I want to wake up in the morning, move through a regular flow of getting ready, choose my clothes, and step into the world feeling like *I think* that woman feels. I used to tell myself I could be like her once I lost 40 pounds, received more education, or made more money. But the truth is far more simple.

Confidence is an attribute that is made up of entirely more than looks, knowledge, or wealth. It is an inner strength that radiates outward, influencing how you are perceived by others. It shines through in how you carry yourself, express your thoughts, and in your overall demeanor. It is an essential component of a naturally healthy and beautiful life.

Because you can't borrow or buy it, it's important to begin by understanding that confidence comes from appreciating your strengths and weaknesses. Not everyone can be the prettiest or the smartest girl in the room, but you can own *who* you are and embrace what you do well. Listen when there is something you can learn and share when you can make someone else's life better.

Confidence is also closely linked to self-care. Self-care often brings to mind bubble baths, massages, and little getaways. It also includes good hydration, consistent sleep habits, simplified skincare, and beauty routines that enhance natural features rather than concealing them. It's also important to exercise regularly and eat a well-balanced diet, which I'll cover in later chapters.

Stay Hydrated: Water is essential for maintaining healthy skin and overall well-being. Drinking enough water helps flush out toxins, keeps your skin hydrated, and contributes to a radiant complexion. Aim for at least eight glasses of water a day to maintain optimal hydration. Pay attention to your thirst and drink more, if necessary.

Prioritize Sleep: Adequate sleep is crucial for maintaining mental and physical health. Lack of sleep can lead to dark circles, dull skin, and increased stress levels. Shoot for 7-9 hours of quality sleep each night to rejuvenate your body and mind. I've discovered it's helpful to go "old-school" by shutting down my electronic devices, reading a paper book, or journaling before bed.

Develop a Skincare Routine: A simple skincare routine tailored to your skin type can work wonders. Cleansing, moisturizing, and using sunscreen are the basic steps to maintain healthy skin. Look for natural skincare products that nourish your skin without harsh chemicals. Remember, products don't have to be expensive to be effective.

Embrace Minimal Makeup: Less is more when it comes to makeup, especially as we age! I've noticed the more I try to cover up, the more my wrinkles stand out! Embrace a natural look that enhances your features rather than hiding them. Focus on a flawless complexion, well-groomed eyebrows, and a pop of color on the lips and cheeks. Avoid heavy foundation, excessive contouring, and harsh eyeliner.

Dress to Express: Your clothing choices can boost your confidence and enhance your natural beauty. Wear clothes that make you feel comfortable and reflect your personal style.

Seek Professional Guidance: If you're struggling with self-acceptance or finding it challenging to embrace your natural beauty, consider visiting a therapist or counselor. Talking through your feelings and experiences with a professional can provide valuable insights and strategies for personal growth.

Surround Yourself with Positivity: Surround yourself with supportive and positive people who uplift your spirit. Cultivate meaningful relationships that encourage self-love and acceptance. Limit exposure to negativity, whether it's in the media or through social interactions.

Confidence is fascinating; you're not born with it and can't buy it. The only way to achieve it is to learn to love yourself and work with what you've got! Confidence isn't a result of wealth, talents, or someone else's opinion but a reflection of inner strength and self-love that stems from embracing who you are.

Wading In: Who is the most captivating woman you know? What makes her that way?

Deep Dive: How can you authentically boost your confidence?

♥

Wonderfully Made

"I praise you, for I am fearfully and wonderfully made. Wonderful are your works; my soul knows it very well."

Psalm 139:14

We live in a world of choices. We have more options than ever and, quite honestly, more than we deserve. We're bombarded by outside influences at every turn, and it's often difficult to feel like you know what's right for you.

Should you follow the latest trends? If it's temporary, cost-effective, and makes you feel good, like a fun hair color or a new pair of boots, I say go for it!

But some of the latest trends are just plain scary, and I feel like women, especially aging, overweight women, are often easy prey. I know so many naturally beautiful women who have fallen prey to influencers, purchasing creams and potions or succumbing to procedures, all in a quest for youth.

For each naturally aging influencer, two are trying to stop the natural aging process by promoting "options."

I have to tell you, I don't like how I look with gray hair, so I color it, but I can change my mind at any time. I don't like the jiggle under my arms, but I can change that too, with a whole-food diet and some resistance training. Will it take longer than surgery? Yes. Is it good for me in a dozen other ways as well? Yes.

There are several ways to feel beautiful, even when you might think you're not:

Find a great dermatologist. I make a regular appointment once a year to check my skin, but I've also consulted her about natural, inexpensive ways to keep my skin from aging rapidly, especially as I'm working on fat loss.

Find a great hairstylist. Nothing can make you feel better faster than a good cut (and maybe a color!)

Visit your dentist regularly. A strong, bright, healthy smile can take years off, and dental health is essential to overall health. Don't skip it.

Find a bra stylist. Lift those girls up! You look younger and trimmer with the right bra. If you are uncomfortable going to a full-service lingerie store, several online options exist! While you're at it, splurge and buy some matching underwear!

Finally… and the most significant boost of all for me: **Invest in yourself.**

"I'll do it when I __________" is one of those phrases I wish I'd charged a nickel for:

"I'll buy new jeans when I reach my goal weight."

"I'll get a cute new haircut when my face is thinner."

"I'll join you in the lazy river when I can fit in a swimsuit."

"I'll splurge on family pictures when I lose 50 pounds."

Live your life! And do the little things that help you feel good about yourself now. The years speed by faster than we can ever hope to control, and it's unfair to yourself AND the people who love you to wait another day to do the things that might just make you happy.

I was likely at my lowest self-esteem in the spring of 2021. My oldest son was getting married, and I felt blah at best. The world had been closed down, so I didn't worry too much about my ashy hair and sloppy clothes, but as things started to open up, I was thrown into a spin of panic.

I imagined people would think poorly of me because I had let myself go. And that's not the case at all, is it? You read those words, and you thought, "Oh my gosh. That poor woman. I bet no one thought anything about what she looked like."

But you've thought it about yourself, haven't you?

I'd heard of House of Color[2] via Instagram, but I didn't know anyone who had gone through the process. I needed a little pick-me-up, so I hesitantly signed up for color analysis, justifying it as necessary before I invested in a mother-of-the-groom dress. Surely, I should look good on one of the most important days of my son's life, right? I was skeptical that the appointment would be worth the cost, but I needed help.

Surprisingly, the knowledge I gained in two short hours was priceless. I left with a palette of colors that made me feel younger, prettier, and more confident. I was a big believer in black clothes (and if I'm being honest, I still kept a couple of my favorite pieces), but I feel so much more like myself in my new autumn palette (which is so much more exciting than the brown and gold you're imagining!).

I followed up last summer with a style consultation. I was nervous, imagining the process of parading around in front of other women in different clothes! It couldn't have been more different. I sent in some measurements and completed a brief questionnaire before the first class. I learned a lot about proportions, lifestyle, and body architecture. And even though I participated with doubt lingering in the back of my brain, I've discovered a wonderful sense of freedom and a renewed appreciation for the clothes in my closet!

I buy the right items now, saving time and money, instead of ordering the wrong clothes and returning them repeatedly. I've sorted my closet and added a few pieces I really love.

House of Colour has been offering Color and Style analysis since 1985. This UK company was founded by image consultant Carolyn Miller, based on color theories developed in the 20th century by artist Johannes Itten. She worked to modify an earlier version of the four-season analysis to incorporate flexibility and individualized results.

House of Colour expanded its offerings to the United States in 2010 and continues growing as new franchise locations open yearly.

The website states, "*While fashions, trends, and fads come and go, the theory of colour, as interpreted by House of Colour, remains based on science, logic, and objectivity, enabling every client to take their individual WOW colours and look and feel wonderful. Your confidence grows, and the journey to empowerment begins!*"

I sat down with three consultants who work together locally to ask them a few questions.

Kim Jensen, the franchisee, and her associates, Jenna Davidson and Krissi Pierce, met me on a cold, snowy day at their office in Ames. They were engaging and friendly and played well off one another. It felt like eavesdropping on girlfriends chatting about work over lunch! As much as I insisted I had the best job (when running the gym), they argued theirs couldn't be beaten.

My first question tried to divide them (but failed): Which is better? Color or Style?

They unanimously agreed both were equally important, and Krissi summed it up nicely: "Color is the missing puzzle piece for many people. It starts with why you like the things you like, but you just can't put your finger on what makes you feel great."

Kim chimed in, "Color is a great start, but style takes it to the next level- it hones in on who you are and how to dress… I think it's easy to buy things in your colors without regard to style and still not feel amazing. Style pulls it all together".

I asked them to simplify the benefits for me. What can *House of Color* offer women?

Confidence: Women report feeling like they've been given permission to wear beautiful colors and fun styles.

Simplicity: When everything in your closet works together and your makeup and jewelry match, you save time and money and reduce stress.

Empowerment: This one surprised me, so I followed up with Jenna after our interview. She works part-time as a House of Color consultant and also as a professor. I instantly thought about "work empowerment," knowing she was a woman teaching at a local college. But her response was gracious, not about anything except her feelings about the service she could provide.

"…I am the type of person who wants to support people and build them up when they are around me. I try to convey that to the client. Each person is uniquely beautiful, and knowing your best colors enhances that beauty. Some of the smallest changes can have the biggest impact on the way someone feels!"

So, my next question: If a woman had fifty dollars to spend on herself, where would she get the biggest bang for her buck? Kim immediately jumped in and said a twenty-five dollar top and a twenty-five dollar lipstick.

Krissi backed her up, "I'd agree on a top in your colors, but I think it also depends on your style. We always tell people to start with what's surrounding their faces first because that's where they have the biggest impact. Get your makeup right and a top in your colors. Those two things would be a huge step in the right direction."

Next, we talked about their clients, and I asked them to share a story that impacted their lives and how they do business. All three had examples of women who shared how they felt more beautiful and confident, and Jenna told a story that touched close to home.

She had a mother-daughter consultation- the mom was in her sixties, and the daughter was close to forty. The daughter was a successful businesswoman and went first. She was excited to learn her power colors. After she finished, her mom sat in the chair. Jenna felt like she probably dragged her feet coming in, agreeing only to make her daughter happy.

"I had just finished doing her colors and makeup and was preparing to take an after photo… I looked up to see tears coming down her face. I put my hand on her shoulder and asked if she was okay. She assured me she was fine but had felt so lost as a sixty-year-old woman. Like society had ignored her because as you get older, people seem to focus less on the elderly."

"She told me she hid in neutral colors- grays, blacks, creams. Sitting here, looking in the mirror, she could finally see who she wanted to be."

Jenna shared how she was recharged and realized their service helps someone for much longer than just one appointment. Many clients told her they spent years living in neutral colors because they didn't want to stand out. "Colors don't necessarily make you stand out. They just make you look your best."

Finally, with the ice broken, I talked about the investment a woman has to make to schedule the consultations. We talked about those of us who were working to lose weight and change our bodies. Should we wait until we're the "right size"?

Kim said, "This is a service you will use every single day for the rest of your life in many different areas. It will save you time, increase your confidence, give you a pep in your step, and help you when you're in the middle of the journey. (It will help) who you are right now, and make that version your very best with colors and style. It's not something dependent on weight loss or gain. It's not dependent on looking better first... it's the current version, the one you are right this second, looking your best."

Jenna said, "And it will continue for the rest of your life. It's not like you're joining a gym, getting a haircut, or doing makeup. It's a one or a two time appointment, and it becomes pennies on the dollar when you realize you'll benefit for the rest of your life.

Krissi added, "This is more about the vanity side of it, but I do feel like everyone should have permission to look in the mirror and feel good about themselves. Everyone has a goal, right? But that doesn't mean you can't look and feel your best until you reach that goal! Even things as simple as wearing my colors when I work out help me feel better about myself, so I actually want to go to the gym. Some might think that's silly, but it motivates me.

I know my colors are my colors forever, but I was curious if my style would change based on my size. I knew a lot of my clothing style would be influenced by my proportions, but I wondered if I were to get to a smaller size, would my style change?

Kim reassured me that my analysis would hold up over time, adding, "If someone's style changes, it's more likely due to lifestyle than size. I've worked with clients, and I told them that when they retire, their style might slide a bit. For example, if you're a classic romantic, you might shift toward a natural romantic when you aren't dressing for work every day. There could be a slight change in that sense based on lifestyle."

"We talk about your body architecture, and your bone structure is not going to change," added Krissi.

Kim shared, "No job compares to the gift of empowering women to love themselves. We say it all the time. We have the best job ever. I decided to go into the area of fashion to help women find the confidence to love who they are and how God made them. That's also why I joined House of Color.

Krissi closed out our interview with hope for women like me who don't necessarily like to shop. "I think at the client level, it's almost more impactful for the women who don't love fashion or style because it gives them the ease of being able to have a closet that really works for them; they don't have to work hard at it, and they don't have to sit and think about following trends."

The cost varies throughout the country, but the short-term investment can give you the knowledge and permission to look your best, no matter how much you weigh or how your body changes, for the rest of your life.

Wading In: What have you been waiting to do "until" you reach your goal?

Deep Dive: How could investing in yourself help you now, in the middle of your journey?

Crowding Out to Simplify Your Look

1 minute:

- Refresh your lipstick- it will make all the difference!
- Sort clothes in your closet by function or color- short-sleeved shirts together, skirts together, or red, blue, and brown.

5 Minutes:

- Perfect a 5-minute make-up routine.
- Refresh your hair- flip upside down and brush or run your fingers through it. Flip back up and shake.
- Remove all clothes that are permanently stained or damaged from your closet.
- Remove seasonal clothes (or move them to the back of your closet).

10 Minutes:

- Toss old make-up.
- Sort! Remove all clothes that no longer fit or you haven't worn in the last six months.

30 Minutes:

- Experiment with a new hairstyle- straighten, curl, or twist it up. Have fun!
- Try on all your clothes and clear out the pieces that don't fit

perfectly. If they are within your goal range- pack them away and label the box so you can "go shopping" when your current clothes are too large.

♥

Chapter 4

Up & Down

Breaking Point

I remember the first time I made a conscious decision to lose weight. Jeff and I had been invited to a wedding, and I wanted to splurge on a new dress. I threw my hair up in a ponytail, removed my stained sweatshirt, grabbed my bag, and headed to the mall.

I went to my favorite department store, and because I lived life in "one size fits all" stretchy leggings and oversized sweatshirts, I was clueless about my current size. I grabbed some of this and a little bit of that and headed into the dressing room. With three-way mirrors all around me, I wiggled, jumped, and danced in and out of several dresses that day. The proverbial fly on the wall would have seen me stand on my tiptoes (if I were 3" taller, I would surely look better in each dress, right?), suck in my stomach, and pivot to look at my backside. There wasn't a dress in that store that hid the fact that I had gained several pounds since my last shopping event. So, I went to the next store, and the next, and the next.

I finally ended up at the last store in the mall. I stood, looking through the display window at a beautiful dress, but it was in the plus-size store. I'd never been in there. It was like a barrier in my brain that said, "No! No, you can't go in there!" And why not? At one point, I'd moved from a children's store to a teen store. Why in the world couldn't I confidently walk into a women's store?

Eventually, my watch crept closer and closer to school pick-up time, and I still didn't have a dress, so I took a deep breath and walked through the doors. With the help of a lovely salesperson, I grabbed three options and found my way to the dressing room. The dresses slipped on and zipped with ease- no shimmying required.

I sat down on the ridiculous little chair they put in the room and cried. I cried because I felt alone. I cried because I felt forgettable. I cried because I found a place where I didn't feel embarrassed and didn't need help getting dressed. I cried because I felt bad about feeling so sad.

I got up from my pity party, bought the dress (and the best bra ever), and headed home. On the way, coincidentally, I heard a commercial for a ten-week weight loss challenge starting at a local gym. I rolled into the garage, left the dress in the car, and signed up before I could change my mind.

That decision and a few others led to a rollercoaster ride of life changes and experiences for me (and my family). I dove headfirst into the program, pushing back the tears first when I had to stand half-dressed in front of a stranger to take my before photos and again every time I couldn't make it through a task. I had reached my breaking point, and nothing was going to stand in my way.

I worked with thousands of women, many of whom joined the gym because they had also reached a breaking point. Embarking on an exercise program is a deeply personal journey and can be triggered by various internal and external factors.

One of the most common motivators is the desire for improved body image. Like me, many women have experienced moments of frustration and self-doubt while shopping for clothes or looking in the mirror. Their self-esteem seems tied directly to their physical appearance. It's rarely about conforming to societal beauty standards but about feeling comfortable in their own skin.

Weight loss often plays a significant role in motivating us to begin an exercise program. There's something about seeing a certain number on the scale that drives us to want to change. Events like weddings, reunions, or milestone birthdays can serve as specific targets for some, spurring them to take action and make lasting changes to their bodies and overall health.

The pursuit of better health is another reason that drives us towards exercise programs. Sometimes, it's the fear of developing health issues or the desire to overcome existing ones. Many of us are inspired to exercise after witnessing the transformations of family members or friends who adopt a healthier lifestyle. Others join, hoping to avoid the diseases that impacted the life of a loved one.

Stress relief and mental well-being are also important factors that encourage women to embrace exercise. The demands of daily life, work, and family responsibilities can create immense stress, and physical activity serves as a powerful outlet. Engaging in exercise releases endorphins, which are natural mood lifters, helping us cope and maintain a positive outlook.

We embark on exercise programs for many reasons, driven by our unique experiences and motivations. I lost several pounds and inches and gained endurance aerobically during the ten-week session.

I felt good. I looked good. And I made many trips back to those stores to shimmy into the dresses I hadn't been able to buy. I told myself I was getting healthier, and I suppose I was improving the health of my heart and lungs and building strong, healthy muscles, but all along, I was establishing new criteria of worthiness. I was completing the story that began in that dressing room.

Big girls are alone. Fit girls have friends. Big girls are forgettable. Fit girls get noticed. Big girls are sad. Fit girls are happy.

Little did I know the impact these thoughts would have on my self-worth in the years to come when I couldn't sustain my weight loss.

Wading In: What was your breaking point?

Deep Dive: How can exercise help you feel better about yourself?

♥

Ground Zero

I still have nightmares of the dreaded step test on Orientation Day. Everyone had to march up and down for two minutes to determine if they were "fit enough" to join a weight loss challenge.

The metronome ticking:

Up.Up.Down.Down.

Up.Up.Down.Down.

Up.Up.Down.Down.

Two ridiculous minutes of dry mouth, heavy breathing. "You can do this".

Heart pumping, quads burning. "Don't stop."

Foot slipping, bile rising. "I'm going to be sick."

Head exploding, hamstrings screaming. "The guy next to me quit… they're leading him away. I can't quit, they have my picture… I have to make it through".

Finally, after what seemed like an eternity, they stopped the timer and told us to sit on the floor. They directed us to find our pulse and count for fifteen seconds.

Ha! Right! I nearly died, and I'm supposed to try to find my pulse?

It wasn't where it was supposed to be. My pulse left my wrist and was hidden in the front of my head, echoing through my ears with a steady thump.thump.thump.

By the time I realized the pounding was my pulse, time was up! I had no idea what my number was! They had my picture, *and* I made it through torture, but I was still going to be kicked out because I couldn't find my pulse!

Next, we were told to rest and record our pulse (take your number and multiply by 4). This just keeps getting better and better, doesn't it? I just made it through a near-death experience, and you want me to multiply the 7432 thumps times 4? I was dying, and I was going to be kicked out. I peeked at my neighbor's stat sheet. She had written down 106. Sounds good… I'm a little older and a little heavier. I wrote down 126. It seemed like a safe bet to me.

I thought we were done, so I rolled over to all fours and prepared to try to stand on very wobbly legs, but I was instructed to stay still. We had to measure our heart rate again… two minutes after the torture ended, my panic attack was still in full mode, and I got to find my pulse again. Wait! Where was that girl? I needed to know her heart rate to calculate mine! Was it supposed to go up after two minutes of rest?? Mine certainly was!

Heart racing, I decided to flat-out lie and wrote down 60. I would find out later in my career that that would have been an athlete level of recovery, not overweight, desk-sitting, middle-aged mother recovery, but they took it, and I made the cut.

Ten weeks flew by. Many of the days were filled with tears, initially when lactic acid surged through my body like wildfire, begging me to quit and then pushing me to feel nauseous when I didn't. The tears also flowed on that glorious day when I didn't feel sick and didn't have to stop. My body was working at its maximum capacity, and I experienced immense satisfaction every time I made it through another task. It was good to know my body was adapting to the challenge and my brain was willing to endure discomfort for the sake of accomplishment.

Looking back, I can't believe I made it through. I started the program from a very deconditioned state- I hadn't worked out for twenty years, and I had recently quit smoking. I like to believe that my body remembered what it was like to be healthy, allowing me to push in ways I'd never pushed before. But the truth is that I was probably lucky.

If you haven't exercised for a long time and feel very out of shape, joining a fitness program can be intimidating. There are some basic ways to begin your fitness journey at home and prepare for a program.

The most important thing is to establish a routine of regular physical activity. You can make a difference quickly, but you have to be faithful to the plan. Start with simple activities like walking or riding a stationary bike. These low-impact exercises will help improve cardiovascular endurance and build a foundation for more intense workouts down the road.

Incorporating bodyweight exercise is another great way to get started. Exercises like squats, lunges, push-ups, and planks can be done at home and require no equipment. They help strengthen muscles and improve your overall stability.

Don't be embarrassed to modify these exercises. They may be basic movements, but they can be hard to do properly if your body is not used to moving that way.

Squat = Chair Sit: Choose a stable chair that's the right height for you to sit with your body at 90° angles (hip to knee to ankle). Place your feet shoulder-width apart and raise to standing. Sit down and repeat ten times. Add additional sets as you feel stronger.

Lunge = Stabilized Reverse Lunge: Stand in a doorway with both hands lightly grasping the casing for balance. Perform a reverse lunge by stepping backward with one leg while keeping the front knee bent and then lowering your body. Alternate and repeat on each side five times. Again, add sets when you can.

Push-up = Wall Push: With your arms fully extended, place your hands on the wall at shoulder level with hands and feet a little more than shoulder-width apart. Holding your tummy muscles tight, slowly bend your elbows until your chin reaches the wall. Then, return to the starting position. Repeat ten times a couple of times a day.

Plank = Dead Bug: Lie on your back with your arms extended toward the ceiling and your feet lifted off the floor with knees bent to 90°. Focus on keeping your back flat on the floor (don't let it arch up) and your core muscles tight. Slowly lower one heel to the floor, then back to the starting position, and repeat on the opposite side. As you build your core strength, you can increase resistance by extending one leg at a time, holding it in place a few inches above the floor for two seconds.

Be patient and kind to yourself. Progress may be slow at first, but consistency is key. Celebrate small victories, and don't be discouraged by setbacks. Every step you take towards a healthier, more active lifestyle is a step in the right direction. Starting from scratch may seem daunting, but with dedication and perseverance, you can prepare your body for a fitness program and achieve remarkable results. You'll discover that your body can adapt to new challenges, and your determination will lead you to a sense of accomplishment you've never known before.

Wading In: How would you describe your current level of fitness?

Deep Dive: Write the ending for your fitness story.

No Pain, No Gain

Once upon a time, long ago, when I was thirteen, I was a state champion swimmer and a 200-yard Individual Medley record holder. I swam every day for several years, sometimes practicing twice a day and competing every weekend. I was a Nervous Nelly at swim meets, bouncing my feet incessantly, nibbling on Knox blocks, and picking at my fingernails until the last race was complete.

I grew up thinking achy muscles and Charley horses in the middle of the night were normal… the price I had to pay for success. I'd stretch, rub out the knots, or walk it off just in time to dive back in the pool.

As I entered my adult fitness era, the aches and pains returned, but my body didn't recover quite as quickly as it did when I was a teenager. Leg day = fear of sitting, and tricep day = top shelf avoidance. I wore my post-workout "waddle" like a badge of honor, knowing there would be no gain without pain.

Once I started coaching, I took this belief to the floor, creating workouts to push my members to their maximum potential day after day. A little more… and a little more! You can do anything!

Unless you can't.

"Good Lord, Kim! Were you trying to kill all of us? Or just me?"

I could count on it almost every day as class was winding down. On mornings when she had to sneak out early for work, I anticipated a text saying the same.

It wasn't uncommon to receive groans and glares as I led a group through a kickboxing class, but very few of my members rewarded me with laugh-out-loud text messages and GIFs later in the day when they were starting to feel the post-workout warmth seeping into their muscles.

Deb walked into the gym for the first time in 2011. She was funny and intelligent, the kind of person you meet and instantly think, "She's wonderful… why didn't I meet her sooner?" She was a faithful journaler, always working on getting her food "just right." She worked out hard but would often stop to take a break or leave the floor unexpectedly. I rushed out after her one day, and she shared that she had a heart condition that caused her resting rate to start at a level that most of us work to reach.

She was exercising, under the guidance of her cardiologist, trying to build her stamina and reduce her meds. Weight loss was a goal, but not the primary one.

Most of us view exercise as a necessary evil to lose weight or prevent gain. Many exercised as children, but that was likely in the name of fun or a sport.

Until I met Deb, I rarely thought about its value in helping reverse the medical blows we receive throughout life. She was acutely aware of what her body could and could not do. She often knew she was "off" before her heart-rate monitor started beeping at her. With consistent exercise and weight management, she was able to reduce her need for a few of her meds and ultimately improve her outlook on life.

Over the years, I have witnessed more people using exercise as medicine. Whether for disease management, stress reduction, preparation for surgery, or recovery, exercise can profoundly affect your health.

My friend Sherri used exercise as a tool to "get herself back" after a well-fought battle against breast cancer. She walked into my gym for the first time after completing her treatment. I didn't know her while she was battling the disease, but I have to believe her attitude was one of the reasons she was victorious.

Exercise was her route back to the life she came from, and she took every day in stride, working out consistently and eating to recover. She won her challenge after making significant physical changes and improving her strength and speed. She has a million-dollar smile and a desire to share the good things she discovers with others. She was undoubtedly the best spokesperson I ever had!

Other people exercise to maintain a life they already love. I'll never forget the day Katie walked in to sign up for personal training. She had been a member since the early days of the gym. Her passion for wellness was infectious, and became an instructor and peer coach.

When she challenged, she was a fierce competitor. I think it was a skill mastered in a household of high-achieving men! Her husband worked out with her, and they raised three sons who became collegiate wrestlers.

She always pushed herself, often logging extra cardio miles throughout the week, but I was also surprised by the desire for extra resistance.

I'm over-simplifying this, but it turned out Katie had a brain tumor. It was non-malignant but growing and needed to be removed. She knew the pros and cons of surgery and also the risks of recovery. Her goal was to be as strong and healthy as possible before the tumor was removed so she could recover quickly and not become a burden to her family. She pushed through headaches and worried about being the best she could be on the day of surgery.

Her hard work and determination prepared her for a better recovery than anticipated. Years later, she continues to prioritize her health and remains one of my greatest sources of inspiration.

As you begin your journey, it's good to let your doctor know you're starting a program. If you're battling a chronic illness or ominous diagnosis, it's imperative. It's also important to track the way you feel along the way:

Listen to your body: If an activity makes you feel different (dizzy, headache, nauseous), find out why.

Surround yourself: Share your space with people who know your goals and limitations.

Be the Boss: Doctors work for you. Don't settle on symptom management. Find someone who will help you determine the cause and work toward your healthy goal. Don't be afraid to interview potential doctors or make a change.

Be excited: Celebrate your non-scale victories.

Share your story: You never know who you might help.

Do new things: Your body is capable of many beautiful things. Find the movement that works best for you.

Wading In: Why do you exercise?

Deep Dive: Read your answer to the question above.
Why do you want that?

Love Yourself

"Love yourself enough to live a healthy lifestyle."

Jules Robson[1]

According to a report on the *Mayo Clinic*[2] website, a healthy adult should get at least 150 minutes of moderate aerobic activity or 75 minutes of vigorous aerobic activity a week (or a combination of the two). Increase that to 300 minutes a week if you want to lose weight (or maintain weight loss).

This is a hard pill to swallow for a lot of people. Many can't find time to relax, much less pack a bag, show up to the gym, work out at the end of the day, and go home to deal with everything else life throws their way.

But even small amounts of physical activity are helpful. Moving can add up, even if only for short periods throughout the day. Examples of moderate aerobic exercise include activities like walking, biking, and swimming, but could also include hiking, mowing the lawn, or playing tag with the kids. Vigorous aerobic exercise could consist of running, High-Intensity Interval Training (HIIT) drills like Tabata sprints, a bodyweight circuit, or, my favorite, ballroom dancing!

You can also mix the two intensities throughout your workout. When I taught kickboxing at my gym, I always tried to maintain a steady pace to warm up and build to a high-energy burn-out phase to spike the heart rates of my gym members.

If you're just getting started, you should exercise in a way you enjoy. The focus should not be on the end goal but rather on tomorrow:

What can I do today that I'll want to do again tomorrow?

Or maybe, if you're starting from a place of recovery:

What can I do today that will allow my body to do it again tomorrow?

I'm a huge fan of walking. Last winter, after years without a regular exercise plan, I made it my mission to research the benefits of a simple walk. Every day for three months, I walked for the sole benefit of enjoyment. I didn't track my heart rate or my steps. I didn't have a "mile goal"- I just walked.

I set my alarm, lured by the promise of sunrise over the ocean rather than fitness. Surprisingly, I didn't miss a day. I faithfully got up, laced my shoes, and moved my body. I know this will shock you: I lost 35 pounds, and my endurance improved.

Start by simply putting one foot in front of the other. You might choose to walk for a time or to a destination. Do it again tomorrow. And the next day. And when it's easy, set the time a little longer or the destination a bit farther.

Your body will tell you when it's ready for more. When that day comes, you have several options to vary your workouts and turn up the intensity: You could consider joining a class like water aerobics or spin. You could head to the gym and jump on a treadmill, an elliptical machine, or a stair-stepper. I like to challenge myself with different times and intensities. You could also check out the options online: Couch to 5K, Tabata, or Low-impact workouts.

Just remember, if you try to go from 0-60 without preparation, there is a good chance something will break. Ease into your workout plan by challenging yourself a little more every day. If things get too hard, lower the intensity by working at half speed or keeping one foot on the ground, sidestep instead of hopping, or raise your arms to shoulder height instead of over your head. The important thing is to move, not necessarily how far you move!

The *Mayo Clinic* Report[3] also recommends strength training for all major muscle groups at least twice a week. Many women seem to think that weight training involves barbells and heavy plates, and although it is fantastic to "lift heavy things," it's not the only way. If powerlifting is your goal, I'd recommend finding a trainer to help you. A quality trainer will ensure you build your strength with proper form to ensure your success comes without injury.

At my gym, we attacked weight training days with resistance bands, kettlebells, and core balls. The rule of thumb was to isolate specific muscle groups and practice three sets of specific exercises with enough weight to "fail" between 8-12 repetitions. You probably had too much weight if you couldn't repeat a motion at least eight times with proper form. If you could sail through twelve reps without noticing you have a weight in your hand, you likely needed more.

Weight machines, resistance bands, and body weight exercises offer many options. Try various exercises with different means of resistance to find which you like best!

It all sounds good in theory, right? But if you're like me (and more than fifty percent of the people who join a gym each year), you know you have to move, but everything else on your plate is more important. You need to get up before the sun rises or drag yourself into the gym at the end of your day… or do you?

During the last few months, I've discovered that I don't really like exercise. Shh! Don't tell anyone, but nothing appeals to me less, except for maybe cleaning the house. So I've decided to do things that don't feel like exercise.

I walk every day, not to burn calories but to be in nature, to work through my problems, and to be with God. I used to try to reach the magical 10,000 steps, and even though I still wear a step-tracking device, I try to focus on simply getting up and out of my chair. I work in the yard, park far away from the store, and set a timer to get up from this manuscript occasionally.

I've made several promises to myself- one is walking. The other is talking to God, so it's very natural for me to combine them. This works for me, and that is all that matters.

Over the next few weeks, I'd like to challenge you to explore your options, figure out what feels good to you, and do something faithfully every day.

You do You. Set a timer to remind you to get out of your chair at least once every hour. Buy a standing desk. Move around your office as you take a sales call. Walk for half of your lunch break. Sign up for a class. Learn to lift, swim, or dance. Do what brings you joy and makes you want to do it again tomorrow.

Wading In: What is your favorite way to exercise?

Deep Dive: What is something new you'd like to try? Research availability in your area and sign up!

♥

Masterpiece

"For we are God's masterpiece. He has created us anew in Christ Jesus, so we can do the good things he planned for us long ago."

Ephesians 2:10

My health journey has been all over the place. I was a typical child, toddling into life when people still let their kids play outdoors. We rode our bikes everywhere and played until dinnertime!

People who know me know I rarely do things halfway. I'm either all in or all out. A free trial often becomes a year-long commitment; testing the water usually means I'm over my head.

My fitness life has been no different. When I was younger, I swam fifty-two weeks a year and often seven days a week. When I decided to quit swimming, I was "done with it." I haven't been in a pool more than a dozen times since.

The next time I picked up exercise was over-shared in the opening words of this chapter; I was thirty-nine, wanted to become healthy, and fell in love with feeling good. I'm confident I wasn't prepared for what would happen in the coming years, but I wanted to share what I learned. I opened a gym, and fitness became my life for the next decade.

Again, when I was done, I was done. Sleeping in, snuggling up with a good book, and a nightly glass of wine became my go-to self-help rituals.

Fast forward several years. At fifty-four, I had gained back all the weight and added a few extra pounds for good measure. I wasn't on any medications but had psoriasis and acute osteoarthritis in my hands. These auto-immune conditions and never-ending fatigue forced me to look at the way I care for myself.

On top of that, my sons were now married and starting their lives in another place. I wanted to be healthy enough to travel to visit and play grandma someday soon.

Good food (and enough of it) is an integral part of jump-starting my metabolism. I know plain water and sleep are crucial to recovery. And I know movement is the catalyst that makes all these other good choices explode.

I also know I need to have patience. I didn't lose strength and pack on pounds overnight. I'm not going to fix it overnight, either. I need to listen to my body because, quite frankly, it's older and compromised.

Everything in me wants to do more in the gym and restrict calories at home. I want to jump on the scale and "verify" my accomplishments… but how ridiculous is that? I'm a fifty-five-year-old woman, and even though that shouldn't limit WHAT I can do, it sometimes puts the brakes on how fast I can do it!!

I've decided I'll move my body every day and care for it with good food and rest.

Six months into my routine, I'm pretty happy and still going strong. Most of the time, I walk outside or stumble through a recorded class, and I have plans to join a gym again soon.

No matter what time the sun rises, it would be easy to stay in my jammies and pour another cup of coffee. But I don't, because I was meant for more.

The negatives: **I ache. I'm tired. I feel uncoordinated. I'm lonely. I'm hungry.**

And the positives: **I ache**… that incredible warm, burn kind of ache that comes from doing good work. I'm **tired**… but sleeping like a champ! **I feel uncoordinated**… but smarter every time I finish a class. My senior brain is working hard to keep up and keep in rhythm! **I'm lonely**… I miss group fitness, but I know I'm never alone. I've settled into a nice prayer routine, and after our chat is over, I dictate the pages you're reading in this book. **I'm hungry**… but I'm active in the kitchen again. I have a great kitchen, and sometimes I forget how much I love to cook.

I'm 100% committed to improving my health. I don't know if slow & steady wins the race, but I'm willing to bet on baby steps for the win.

Wading In: Why do you want to be healthy?

Deep Dive: What BIG goal is on your fitness bucket list?

♥

Use it or Lose It

I've learned over the years how much I take for granted when it comes to my body. I feel like I used to be invincible! Faster than a speeding bullet! More powerful than a locomotive! Able to leap tall buildings… wait, my mistake– that was Superman.

Let's start over… I used to be young. Able to rebound after a tumble. Able to stumble over a curb without falling to the ground. Able to "hold it" for a few more miles. All of a sudden, I'm not just worrying about cellulite and a tummy pooch. I'm worried about exercising without aggravating my knee or lifting the grocery bags without tweaking my back.

How often have you heard, "It's all part of getting older"?

I get this almost every day from my husband. (who is ancient compared to me- a whopping six years my senior!) I certainly want to age, but I don't think it should have to be quite so painful!

When I was younger, I focused all my efforts on cardio and strength training, using exercise to manage my weight and look the way I wanted.

Today, it has become something completely different, a lifeline of sorts, to the way I want to finish my years.

The *National Institute on Aging*[4] expands the list of beneficial movements to include Balance and Flexibility. As much as it kills me to be reading articles written by an organization created to support an aging population, I'm glad I made it to the point in life where I need it.

Even simple balance exercises, like standing on one foot while you brush your teeth or heel-to-toe walking, can help prevent a tumble. If you know someone who's experienced a bad fall, you likely agree it's worth preventing. My balance was never better than when I focused on resistance and weight-bearing exercises. But true balance work takes more than strong legs and a tight core.

I participated in Tae Kwon Do when my boys were younger and enjoyed the high-energy workout that also helped significantly with my flexibility, so I thought I'd try the "older persons" martial art. I signed up for Tai Chi last year, thinking it would be just a more accessible form of the same movements I learned in the past, but I couldn't have been more wrong.

Tai Chi involves so much control! I had difficulty moving my body slowly and precisely while simultaneously focusing on my breath. The movements were awkward, and my feet or hands were always in the wrong place, but the more I practiced, the better I felt. My heart rate was rarely elevated, but I still experienced that good muscle burn a few hours after class. It's amazing how many muscles I engaged trying to balance myself in a new way!

I'm not sure when I lost my balance and flexibility. I had it in my forties… I know I did. But now it seems like every day I wake up, I'm suddenly uncomfortable doing something I've done my whole life.

I walked last week with my friend while her son had soccer practice. I hadn't seen her for a while, and it was a beautiful day, so I didn't hesitate to join her when she texted the invitation. We enjoyed the warm, sunny day as the kids ran around chasing a ball. As the end of practice neared, the coach called the boys in for a quick meeting. He kneeled on the ground while the players squatted at his level.

I wonder how long it's been since I felt comfortable in that position. It's not that my body can't get there. It just doesn't feel good there. It's amazing what we take for granted. Simple things like touching your toes or looking over your shoulder, squatting or sitting body basic style seem to be there one day and gone the next!

Regular stretching can improve flexibility, but I don't think to do it unless I've "officially" exercised. It's hard to believe that something so easy can greatly impact our quality of life, yet very few people take the time to do it. There are a few important tips before you go gangbusters with your routine:

- Stretch when your muscles are warmed up.
- Stretch after all exercise (even walking or balance training).

- Stretch only far enough to feel a slight pull, never so far that it hurts.
- Breathe normally while holding a stretch.

I'm feeling pretty good about myself after a winter of walking and stretching and doing good things for my body. There are things I can do now that I thought I'd lost the ability to do forever, like touching my toes and jogging up a flight of stairs. Every week that passes, I notice more endurance, and that motivates me to continue.

In a never-ending quest to learn more about my body and right the wrong, I signed up for a class to strengthen my pelvic floor. After all, what good is it to be able to walk five miles again if I have to clench my thighs as I run-waddle to a kybo or squat behind a tree before I get home?

Several of us met for a three-week class, so obviously, the problem was not exclusively mine. It was taught by Amy Ralston, a licensed Physical Therapist Assistant specializing in Prenatal and Postpartum Corrective Exercise.

During the first class, we learned about the structure of the pelvic floor, its function and importance, and the causes of dysfunction. During the second class, we learned about core activation, and in the final class, we learned about hip strength. The course was informative and incredibly helpful; I wonder how many other "old age issues" could be turned around with proper care and training of the surrounding systems.

I asked Amy a few follow-up questions after completing the course. She is currently a women's health personal trainer, teaching courses on pelvic floor health. She chose to work in this field because there is a massive need for people specializing in women's health in the medical and fitness world. "Most women I know have dealt with or are dealing with some sort of pelvic floor issue. Whether that's pain, incontinence, or prolapse, there are many dysfunctions. Everyone should know how to use their bodies and their pelvic floor correctly."

She indicated that it's mostly about education and prevention for the younger generation. The goal would be a solid and functional core and pelvic floor to prevent issues down the road.

"In terms of pregnant or postpartum women, this (pelvic floor training) can be significantly important. Training can help moms-to-be have an easier pregnancy, with less pain and hopefully an easier birth process."

She said it's also crucial for women to learn how to start gradually increasing their strength while keeping their bodies safe and avoiding straining during the postpartum period.

She noted that many older women had issues they've been dealing with for years, but it doesn't mean things can't improve. "I have seen women of all ages and sizes improve their symptoms. Unfortunately, I feel like the older population has been taught about the pelvic floor incorrectly. So many women have to retrain their brains and establish a good mind-body connection."

But Kegels help everything, right?

She laughed and said that although that's what most of us have learned, Kegels are not the cure-all most women think.

"Kegels are a strengthening exercise for the pelvic floor, but what if a woman has a tight pelvic floor? That would be like telling someone with a tight neck to hike their shoulders up over and over again. The movement would make their neck pain feel worse, right? It's the same thing. If you are dealing with a lot of tightness, we would work on ways to help relax and unload the pelvic floor."

She noted most of the women she has treated had a tightness issue, which can cause incontinence issues as much as weak muscles.

Her treatment protocol starts with correct breathing techniques to establish good mobility and stimulation of the pelvic floor. "Once they have achieved better mobility, we can start safely incorporating strength training," she said.

I asked Amy what one thing she'd like to teach all women: "How to breathe correctly! Our bodies are built like a pressure system, so when we inhale, our diaphragm contracts downward, increasing pressure on our abdominal structures in our pelvic floor. When we inhale, our pelvic floor should relax down, and when we exhale, it should recoil back to its resting position."

She continued sharing that many women think belly breathing is the same as diaphragmatic breathing. In class, she taught us about "360 breathing" - trying to focus on the belly moving, but the rib cage, and the lower back as well. She indicated it is the best way to get the pelvic floor to relax.

She concluded by sharing that women should know they have options.

"They shouldn't have to settle in terms of pain, whether that's back pain or some type of pelvic pain. They shouldn't have to continue to deal with prolapse or incontinence. There are lots of resources available now that can help women feel their best, not be embarrassed, and improve their quality of life."

She recommends pelvic floor physical therapy. She's been helping clients for the past five years and has seen tremendous results for women of all ages. She added personal training can be an excellent resource for women who need support on how to move their bodies and use them correctly and healthily.

Wading In: What ailment or annoyance could you improve with a trainer?

Deep Dive: Make the call- schedule a consultation with a personal trainer today.

♥

Crowding Out for Movement

1 minute:

- Box Breath

  Breathe in… 1…2…3…4

  Hold…1…2…3…4

Breathe out…1…2…3…4

Hold… 1…2…3…4

Repeat twice

- Body Break! Walk around the office or jog in place.
- Burst! 20 Jumping Jacks or 10 squat jumps.
- Stretch! Stand up, touch your toes, raise your arms above your head, turn your neck from side to side.

5 Minutes:

- Tabata! Set a timer for 20 seconds "on" 10 seconds "rest." Pick any exercise and repeat the series 10 times.
- Body Break! Walk around the office.
- Google 5-minute desk workout- there are some good ones!

10 Minutes:

- Brisk Walk
- Hall Lunges

30 Minutes:

- Walk Outside
- Stretch or Yoga

Chapter 5

Savor

I Can't Eat That!

"I can't eat that!"

If I had a nickel for every time I heard that phrase as a coach, I'd be wealthy beyond my wildest dreams!

I've seen and heard (and tried) it all: no carb, low carb, low fat, and low calorie. I've counted calories, weighed every morsel, and choked down more shakes than I'd care to think about. Every plan worked for a while until I burned out on veggies and egg whites and starved myself through my workouts.

Chances are, if you're a woman in the twenty-first century, you've also experienced this.

I'm thrilled to share that I've reached a point in my life when I've started to regain the pleasure of eating. No, this doesn't mean I've resigned to being overweight. It means I've had to think about how I view food.

For as long as I can remember, food has had a label that comes with either acceptance or guilt:

Good-Bad, Fast-Slow, Whole-Manufactured, Healthy- Unhealthy. Clean- Dirty.

I've worked with hundreds of people who prided themselves that they hadn't eaten bacon or bread in years. They've learned to control their cravings by hiding the chocolate chips in the freezer (in a corner, under the chicken, behind the broccoli). They spent years avoiding entire food groups and feeling guilty when they allowed a forbidden morsel to cross their lips. This deprivation lifestyle has caused so many healthy people to not only "fall off the wagon" but to nose dive down a deep, dark cavern of guilt.

I'll be the first to admit that I became one of those wagon slippers. I caught the "get healthy" bug as I was nearing forty and pushed it to the extreme. I exercised six days a week, waking long before dawn so nothing would get in my way. I refused to stay in my warm bed, even on vacation. I balanced my plate and pushed away treats. I looked at foods like corn and potatoes as "bad" and faithfully placed spinach and broccoli on my daily plan. I allowed myself fruit only before 3:00 pm. I bought two different kinds of meat for dinner: marbled, delicious cuts of beef for my guys and chicken breast for myself. I became so obsessed with eating "right" that I always cooked extra food for myself so I wouldn't get caught and have to eat food that I made for them.

I lost weight. And it was fun to slip into smaller clothes and to receive compliments, but it was work, a lot of work, and the food got boring. Night after night (after night) of chicken and lettuce and water-rich vegetables. Sure, I tried to spice it up. Mrs. Dash can fix anything, right? But in the end, I fell off the wagon of good health in favor of variety and flavor.

Fast forward a couple of years, I was going through the motions, talking the talk and helping others, but I had completely given up on my most important client: Me. I was unhappy, several pounds over my "feel good weight," and frustrated with my inability to "fix" myself.

One day, I had a great "back & forth" with a friend about food, exercise, and impossible plateaus. Later, I realized that good health doesn't have to be black or white. There is so much good in the gray zone.

Can I order pasta but choose the lunch-size portion?

Could I put half & half in my coffee occasionally and eat ribeye instead of another piece of chicken?

Is it okay if I make my favorite cake AND eat a piece for no reason?

Could I have potatoes for dinner?

What I've discovered is the answer is always a resounding YES!

Yes, I can live in the gray zone *and* progress toward my goals. I learned that cake and potatoes have a place in my healthy life just as much as tuna and kale. And I know disappointment has ruined more diets than any hot fudge sundae ever dreamed about! I don't indulge often, but when I do, I make sure every bite is worth it! Miraculously, ridding myself of guilt and boredom has lightened the load more than any gluten-free, dairy-free, shake-it-up-and-go plan has in my entire adult life. I'm enjoying meals *and* on my way to a healthier weight.

Most of us spend our lives searching for the magic that will keep us trim, healthy, and confident forever. The truth is there is no perfect diet. There's sound science and a world of ingredients to mix into the "recipe" to make your meals delicious and "good for you." Once you master how to combine Proteins, Carbs, Fats, and Vegetables in ratios and portions that make you thrive, you won't want to eat any other way. Sure, you'll have a treat sometimes, but an occasional treat will not affect your health or the scale if your diet is typically based on whole foods.

My goal is to empower you to reconnect with your body's signals, enabling you to self-coach and guide yourself back on course.

I want you to know:

- you're hungry because your stomach is growling.
- you're "under-carbed" because your workout wasn't great.
- you didn't drink enough water because you can't focus during the day.
- you can't move your ring because of too much salt.
- you're craving sweets because you skipped a meal (or it was too low fat).

I want you to feel so good every day that you sense when something's different and automatically know what's wrong and why. And most importantly, I want you to know how to return to feeling good.

Wading In: Write down what you eat.
No pressure. No expectation. Just write it down.

Deep Dive: Reflect on how each meal made you feel.

♥

In Touch

I'd like to ask you to indulge me for a second to share a story that seems unrelated to my book… And here we go. I introduced you to my son Sam in an earlier chapter. When he was born, he was very sick, and through medical intervention and answered prayers, he survived.

But there was something else that helped to heal his poor little body: my body. My body knew he was premature and sick; therefore, it produced a different formulation of breast milk than it would have if he had been born at full term.

According to a post on the *Stanford Medicine Children's Health* website[1], milk produced by the mother of a preterm baby has more fat, protein, minerals, sodium, chloride, and iron than the milk of a full-term child. It also has higher levels of specific anti-infective properties.

Why do I share this? Because I want you to think for a moment about how incredible our bodies are. They were made to grow, heal, adapt, and know what is best for us.

When we are newborns, we sleep, cry, eat, poop, and repeat. Our decision-making isn't developed enough to overrule our needs, and if we're lucky, someone takes care of those needs promptly, and we are happy.

Somewhere in the first year, our parents get tired of our schedule not being in sync with theirs, and they start to stretch the time between feedings, or they listen to the wisdom of the great aunts and sneak a little bit of cereal into the mix to get us to sleep a little longer. Months turn into years, and eventually, we are forced to satisfy our needs (our hunger) within the limits of another's rules, or we learn to "be hungry" or "behave" when a treat is offered.

We are born as intuitive eaters, following cues of hunger and satiety, but it's easy in this busy, emotional, over-scheduled world to flip those switches off.

As I've shared, I believe our bodies are incredible machines, but to heal and work the way they were created, you often have to reset your thinking and develop new habits.

In their life-saving book, *Intuitive Eating*[2], authors Evelyn Tribole, M.S., R.D. and Elyse Resch, M.S., R.D., F.A.D.A. outline steps to reawaken a more instinctive path back to health. Several of their principles have become mainstays in my view of health, such as honoring hunger, making peace with food, respecting your body, and exercising to feel better.

For some individuals, these steps can be as simple as creating a new routine, changing an everyday habit, or setting a goal.

For others, attempting to make changes can trigger an emotional or physical response. If you find yourself preoccupied with food or your weight, feel guilt or shame in response to a food choice, or find yourself engaging in restrictive measures, I'd encourage you to reach out to a registered dietician or licensed professional counselor. There are incredible healthcare professionals who can help you on your journey towards a healthier life.

If you aren't sure you need help, online resources can provide you with a starting place. Good information and connection to others who may be experiencing some of the same thoughts and feelings can give clarity and direction. A great place to begin is *N.E.D.A.*, the National Eating Disorders Association[3]. The website offers a screening tool, informative blog posts, forums, online links, and a helpline.

Eating and over-exercising disorders are not exclusively teenage and young adult concerns like many of us may think. I've worked with hundreds of amazing women at the gym. I've talked a lot about the ones who made healthy progress and a little about some who gave up on their health goals. But beautiful, strong, healthy women also slipped into a state of "wanting more" and pushed themselves to extreme measures. They often received accolades from others for their ability and work ethic. I'm sad to say I, too, praised them for their discipline, not knowing I was fueling harmful habits.

I'm not qualified to discuss various causes and treatments for these disorders, but there are ways to be caring and supportive of yourself and others.

In a conversation with my friend Roberta Deppe, a Licensed Professional Counselor, I became aware of the seemingly innocent words used in the health and wellness community that can trigger negative responses regarding body image and health. I asked her to read my nutrition and exercise chapters, looking for sensitive issues or potential triggers. I was surprised when she shared about the psychological response a few innocently placed words can have on a person.

In my coaching practice, I quit using terms such as good or bad but didn't think twice about the word clean. Is it the opposite of clean eating or dirty eating? I stopped using the words skinny and fat but never thought about the fact that once a person lost weight, I made sure to tell them I thought they looked beautiful. Were they NOT beautiful before? I quit posting images of how many jumping jacks it takes to burn various kinds of Halloween candy, but I didn't think twice before telling myself, "Earn it" when planning a night out. Now, I work hard to speak affirming words to myself and others: You look so healthy! Great outfit! I love your smile! I feel good!

In the introduction, I asked you to trust me and to work through this book in order. I did so because I've identified ways to right some unhealthy wrongs throughout my journey back to health. I've inflicted a great deal of expectation and disappointment on myself over the fifty-plus years I've lived on this planet, and it's now time to offer myself a bit of love.

Until now, I've asked you to find time to pray, write, and move your body. All these motions bring us here with a greater awareness of what we want and need to live a joy-filled life. Hopefully, you have a "feel goal," and you've begun to get in touch with your body over the last few weeks. Self-awareness and love make you want to be healthy. Recording allows you to identify opportunities. Exercise makes you hungry. Hunger makes you want to eat. Eating makes you feel satisfied. Sleep allows you to heal and to do it all again, day after day.

It's okay to want to lose weight, but lose it because you want to be healthy and be able to do more things. It's okay to want to look different, but choose that too within the lens of self-love. You are wonderful. You are beautiful. You were gloriously made- today, tomorrow, and in all the days to come.

Wading In: Do you view food as "good" or "bad"? If so, when did you start?

Deep Dive: Get in touch with your body. What do you need today?

Convenience

"Everything that lives and moves about will be food for you. Just as I gave you the green plants, I now give you everything."

Genesis 9:3 NIV

There's a good chance this section will bring me the most heartburn and negative comments, but I feel like it's one of the most important topics in the book. Please consider what I have to say and implement what you want to change, or evaluate what I have to say, dismiss it, and carry on the way you have been. It's your choice to think about it and use it as you will. No judgment on my part, ever.

Deep breath… and here we go.

I believe our generation's most significant health problems come from what we put in our bodies. In my lifetime, we have seen fast cooking methods become the norm, and ultra-processed foods have risen to a point where they are now reported to make up 60% of all calories consumed in the United States.

It's essential to recognize that not all processed foods are bad. Many healthy foods have been altered from their original form to become more palatable or more accessible to eat: Dried beans must be cooked, grains need to be processed, and dairy can become a multitude of healthy things, like yogurt, cottage cheese, and even ice cream.

Ultra-processed foods, on the other hand, would include soft drinks, frozen convenience foods like nuggets and pizzas, sweetened breakfast cereals, hot dogs, flavored coffee creamers, and energy drinks. Typically, ultra-processed foods are created with unpronounceable ingredients and may be high in fat and sugar or void in calories, fat AND sugar… How does that work?

With the increased consumption of these easy meals, very few Americans reach the minimum guidelines for recommended foods. According to a 2010 report from the *National Cancer Institute*[4] on the status of the American diet, three out of four Americans don't eat a single piece of fruit in a given day, and nearly nine out of ten don't reach the minimum recommended daily intake of vegetables.

Our bodies were created to respond to *real* food and pure, unadulterated water. Case after case proves the increased health benefits of eating an unprocessed, whole-food diet.

Unfortunately, I know several women my age who haven't learned how to cook the traditional way. Many of us grew up with both parents working full-time jobs. In 1930, only twelve percent of married women had jobs outside their homes. By 1970, fifty percent of single women and forty percent of married women participated in the labor force. By the early 1990s, over seventy percent of women between the ages of twenty-five and fifty-four worked outside the home.[5]

The very real pressures of both adults working outside jobs paved the way for the convenience food revolution. Imagine the gift of an hour and the peace of mind achieved by popping a ready-to-heat meal in the microwave. Or consider the relief from a picky toddler's whining at the end of a long work day by zapping a bowl of mac & cheese instead of fighting over uneaten vegetables.

I get it. I swear I do, but I believe with all that I am, we were not meant to eat things produced in a factory as often as we do. I'm not an expert, but let's take a look at some disturbing trends that have occurred since the convenience food revolution occurred:

- The rate of *ADHD* has increased yearly since 1997 (the first year a national parent survey was offered).[6]
- *ADHD* diagnoses among adults are growing four times faster than diagnoses among children in the United States (26.4% increase among children compared to 123.3 percent among adults)[7,8]
- *Autism* was once a rare disability; in 1970, two (or less) of every 10,000 U.S. children was diagnosed. Today, that number has risen to 1 in 44 U.S. children.[9]
- The prevalence of diagnosed diabetes continues to increase; in 2015, 23.4 million people had been diagnosed with *diabetes*, compared to only 1.6 million in 1958.[10]
- *Obesity* has nearly tripled in the United States over the last fifty years.[11]
- A study by researchers from Brigham and Women's Hospital reveals that the incidence of early onset *cancers* — including breast, colon, esophagus, kidney, liver, and pancreas — has dramatically increased around the world, with the rise beginning around 1990. They report, "From our data, we observed something called the birth cohort effect. This effect shows that each successive group of people born at a later time — e.g., a decade later — have a higher risk of developing cancer later in life, likely due to risk factors they were exposed to at a young age..."[12]
- Environmental and lifestyle factors such as smoking, excessive alcohol intake, and obesity can affect fertility. In addition, exposure to environmental pollutants and toxins can be directly toxic to gametes (eggs and sperm), resulting in their decreased numbers and poor quality, leading to *infertility*, according to the World Health Organization.[13]

You can read various articles about the reasons for the increases, including efficiency in testing and over-diagnosis. Still, the coincidence of the timing of the convenience food revolution and the increase of our various national health crises are too apparent to ignore.

You might argue that I'm a generation off, but consider that we (people born between the late 1960s and 70s) were the first to eat and drink "pretend food" regularly. Heck, I remember the celebration in our house when the Radar Range arrived, complete with the special tray for cooking bacon and the plastic yellow cone that could magically cook popcorn without oil. We cooked entire meals in the microwave oven and did it often because our overworked parents felt good about putting a hot meal on the table after a long day at work. Our moms' guilt for not being as good as their mothers was relieved by the magic of manufactured food cooked in plastic in record time.

It's not their fault for choosing this option, and it's not our fault for eating these foods or continuing the process with our children because we didn't know. But as the third generation of children continues to spiral helplessly out of control, we have to look at the obvious. We have to get back to real food cooked in traditional ways.

I'm not trying to make anyone feel guilty. Unrealistic pressures are put on us daily as we make our way through this life, and I'm not here to make it worse. But I will tell you, there is a better way to shop and cook and eat, a way that will eventually heal our bodies, lose unnecessary weight, and thrive. We have to return to food that is whole, nourishing, *and* convenient.

con•ven•ience- noun

1. the quality of being convenient; suitability.
2. anything that saves or simplifies work, adds to one's ease or comfort.
3. a convenient situation or time; at your convenience

   -adjective 1. easy to obtain, use, or reach; made for convenience.

Please notice it didn't say:

1. Do NOT remove the plastic. Cook according to directions.
2. Open the can and reheat.
3. Pull up to the speaker and order.

Friends, we're all busy. Some of us are juggling the kids' schedules and work or a demanding boss and a fun-loving group of friends. Others are suffering health issues or financial setbacks. But with practice, you can learn to put healthy meals on the table consistently. When I get in a time crunch, I pick up a rotisserie chicken and a bag of salad mix or frozen veggies! Real food cooked by someone else still counts; always remember that!

Most of the meals at my house are created from foods purchased, prepped, and cooked on the weekend. I spend a few hours once or twice a week creating wonderful, delicious, **convenient** foods like hard-boiled eggs, grilled meats, and sliced vegetables.

I eat great meals all week because food is ready to heat and eat! I'm not bored because I don't plan just another "chicken meal." I can open the fridge and decide what I feel like because a variety of food is ready to go.

Pick the protein. Pick a side. Hot or cold? "Toss it in a skillet or throw it on a salad" is often the hardest decision I make after 6 pm.

Another advantage to pre-cooking is that I don't have to rely on supplements for my snacks. How about a slice or two of pork loin and an apple for an afternoon snack? It's entirely more satisfying than a protein bar!

I'd like to challenge you to change your life for a few weeks.

- Change it by rethinking your view of convenience.
- Change it by focusing on how your body feels and what it means to be healthy.
- Change it by realizing that healthy living doesn't just happen Monday-Friday.
- Change it by recommitting to real food and water.
- Change it by claiming the gifts given to us at the beginning of time.

Wading In: Pick one convenience food you rely on daily. What will you replace it with?

Deep Dive: Think about one convenience food you won't give up. What makes it worth the risk?

♥

Discipline Fatigue

"We're told to muster discipline and self-control all day, every day. But discipline is like a muscle and muscles fatigue."

Blue Zones American Cookbook by Dan Buettner[14]

So, I'm going to jump down from the soap box I was perched on because as much as I believe we should eat real food, I also think we need to acknowledge that we can't be perfect.

My observation, after years of low-calorie or low-carb diets, was that I could indeed lose weight, but I was unable to sustain the loss. I tried to live a life sitting outside of celebrations, avoiding birthday cake or a glass of champagne. During holiday gatherings, I refrained from indulging in my favorite traditional dishes, like whipped potatoes with gravy or custard pie. There was even a time when I was so messed up I would take my own food when we attended football parties or family picnics. Now, don't get me wrong, there is nothing wrong with that if you're feeding an infant or if you have an allergy; if you're simply dieting, you should learn to enjoy all foods in limited quantities on your journey to better health.

I don't think it's always okay to eat whatever you want all the time. We have a responsibility to ourselves and those who love us to be healthy. But I do think it's okay to enjoy life, to enjoy food, and to not be afraid to eat something that brings you joy once in a while.

Discipline seems to be the biggest hurdle for most of us. It's the one thing that most health and wellness influencers will tell you matters the most- they seem to wear their discipline as a badge of honor:

Just do it! Be tough! Be strong! Plan to win!

These are great motivations if used occasionally, but typically, these thoughts turn into mantras of shame.

Yesterday, I decided to poll my followers. I asked them what foods or drinks pulled them most easily off their diet plan. Overwhelmingly, the culprits were chocolate and wine. The sad thing is chocolate and wine are not bad, but because those women view the consumption of these foods as failing, they never take their place in a healthy diet. They remain forbidden foods, whispering from the cupboard, making us feel weak.

From my point of view, the misplaced opinion that deprivation is the same as discipline is the reason diets fail, and most women give up trying to change. It's healthy to treat yourself once in a while without worry or shame. You should walk away from extreme restrictions and unrealistic timelines forever. Yes, forever.

You are beautiful and perfect just the way you are. If you want to look different, do something about it in a way that respects all that you are. Treat yourself like a friend would treat you. Look at yourself the way a lover would look at you. Make changes that allow you to be who you want to be for the rest of your life.

I know there are times when there is no way you can think about anything except survival. If you are like me, you're caring for others and moving through your life on a schedule you don't necessarily create. Believe it or not, I've known hundreds of women who have walked away from their plan amid progress because they felt they were fighting a losing battle.

I've spent most of my life as my own worst enemy, setting unrealistic expectations and punishing myself for food slip-ups by doing workouts I didn't enjoy. I told my challenge members, "You can't outwork a bad diet," but I attempted daily to cover up my occasional transgressions with more work. I'd hear stupid things in my head like "calories in, sweat out" as I punched a bag, and eventually, I grew to resent the facade I was trying to uphold. Rather than modify my diet to include the foods I craved, I threw in the towel like many other women I know.

You can only pretend to be perfect for so long- eventually, desire sneaks out from its prison and sabotages your hard work. To prevent a freefall back to your old ways, build new habits that include foods formerly known as forbidden and challenge yourself to not call them cheat foods. They are treats. They have their place in a healthy diet, and you do not have to earn them.

There are times in your life when everything will be going well, then, out of the blue, you get smacked square in the forehead with a roadblock. Maybe you're facing a deadline at work, or a family member is sick. Maybe you're the one who's sick, or you just don't have the energy to think about prepping and planning and balancing your plate. Maybe you're on the vacation of a lifetime, and you just want to follow the crowd. It happens to all of us at one point or another, and usually, that's when you decide to give up. Instead, I'd challenge you to throw your hands up and say, "I give… for now". Stay on track the best you can- balance your convenience store bag of chips with a piece of string cheese and an apple. Or grab a sub; double the protein and add some veggies. Or simply eat what feels right and good at the time, honoring yourself with a bit of grace.

When you fall off track (and you will), my best advice is to shake it off. I know you'll be fine, but because I've lived with the worry myself, I'd like to give you a few tricks to get out of your own way and back in control of your health.

STAY OFF THE SCALE! You already know you feel bloated and sludgy, so why add insult to injury? Wait a few days when you're feeling a little more like yourself.

Balance your plate. Start as soon as possible, maybe with your next meal? I know you probably haven't cooked for the week yet, but you can do it if you have eggs or leftover meat and fruits or veggies. If you have nothing in the fridge, truck your tush to any drive-through and grab a grilled chicken salad. Get vinaigrette on the side because they usually give you too much. Order a burger with extra veggies and less sauce, share the fries, and skip the soda.

Eat regular meals. If you need to, set the alarm on your phone to get you back on track. Check in with yourself when the alarm goes off.

Am I hungry? Am I tired? Do I feel great? It's okay to eat a little bit a few times a day. It's also okay to eat a full meal.

Flush your body. Dump the cold coffee (or warm diet Coke) from your cup and guzzle some water. You know you can see the zipper mark from your jeans furrowed in your belly because of the salt you consumed. Flush it out. Get at least 80 ounces in today and tomorrow.

Move. You may or may not feel like working out. If you're suffering from a food coma, go for a walk. If you're in the mood to go to the gym, honor the urge to move your body. You know you'll feel better!

Catch up. You have a lifetime to catch up on emails and phone calls. Take some time to wind down after a long day. Read, write, or curl up and simply be with your people. Go to bed early and set your alarm for the last moment to get ready without rushing.

Rinse and repeat. Care for yourself as many days as necessary to feel back in the groove.

Look at yourself. Love yourself.

Give yourself the grace you would offer your most loved one and learn what works for you.

Grace is never earned- simply given.

Wading In: How did you love someone today?

Deep Dive: How did you love yourself today?

♥

What's On Your Plate?

Grocery shopping when I owned the gym was always an intimidating event for me. I never failed to bump into gym members when I bought frozen pizzas for the boys and their friends or a few bottles of wine for a dinner party. They would talk to me, but they rarely looked at me. They were always looking in my cart! I started to feel guilty and found myself sneaking to the store before the first light of day to get in and out if I wanted to buy something others would consider bad. I tried to reinforce the "no food is bad food" mantra with my challengers, but deep down, I knew they didn't buy in because I didn't believe it myself.

Although there's no perfect diet, I believe there is a perfect diet for each of us. So many of us spend our lives searching for the easy solution, the pill or potion or macro ratios that will make it easy to reach our goals. According to the *Boston Medical Center*[15], an estimated 45 million Americans go on a diet each year, and we spend a staggering $33 billion on weight loss products annually. Unfortunately, few of us are patient enough to put in the time or effort to see results, no matter what we do. Many people start a new diet and expect results within a matter of days. We believe the initial change on the scale is fat loss, when it's usually water weight, and when we plateau after a week, we try to convince ourselves we must be building muscle.

The truth is there is no magic: the fat will come off, and the muscle will grow, but just as we gained weight over time, it will take time to change.

Our bodies are incredible! We were created to respond to macronutrients (protein, fat, and carbohydrates) in their natural form as ways to sustain us or even help us improve our health. Every person should experiment to find the perfect ratio to make their bodies thrive. Each kind of nutrient provides something essential for our bodies.

Protein is so critical it's often called the building block of life. Every cell in the human body contains this macronutrient. You need protein to help your body repair cells and make new ones. These foods are broken down into parts called amino acids during digestion. The human body needs a number of these amino acids and enough of them to maintain good health. Amino acids are found in animal sources such as meats, milk, fish, and eggs. They are also found in plant sources such as soy, beans, legumes, nut butter, and some grains (such as wheat germ and quinoa).

Dietary fats are essential for maintaining good overall health, especially as you age. Fat is necessary for proper brain function. Omega 3 fatty acids are the essential building blocks of our brain, and they're important for learning and memory. Fat also helps give your body energy, protects your organs, supports cell growth, controls cholesterol and blood pressure, and helps your body absorb vital nutrients. It slows digestion, keeping you full longer. Healthy fat is found in certain fish, nuts, seeds, egg yolks, avocados, and cold-pressed oils.

Finally, carbohydrates provide the fuel that keeps us running. Foods high in carbohydrates are an important part of a healthy diet. They provide the body with glucose, which is converted to energy used to support bodily functions and physical activity. Carbohydrate quality is important, and some carbohydrate-rich foods are better than others. The best carbohydrates are found in fruits, vegetables, and whole grains. Unfortunately, our palettes have become attuned to highly refined carbohydrates like white bread, tender pastries, sugary cereal, and pasta.

I spent a lot of years restricting myself. As I banned the "bad," it seemed like I craved those foods more than ever. Journaling helped me discover which foods made me feel good and which made me feel crummy. Today, I find it empowering to be in control: If I want it, I eat it. I know how to balance my plate so I don't experience highs and lows all day, and my cravings have all but gone away.

If more of us would take time to track our food, pay attention to how we feel, and limit the foods that cause us dietary distress, we could reduce many ailments that keep us from thriving.

It's important to emphasize healthy food does not have to taste bland or be expensive. Your meals don't have to consist of plain lettuce salads with baked chicken breasts and steamed broccoli (although I think those things are delicious). You can create incredible meals that let you enjoy your new, healthier lifestyle. Food can be nutritious, delicious, and combined in a way to make your body feel perfect.

Healthy eating means many things to many people. Look at the cookbooks and diet plans to hit the bookshelves every year, not to mention the countless number of supplements, pills, and potions on the market. There is a good reason why nutrition is one of my priorities. If you master nutrition, everything else falls into place. Someone once told me, "You can exercise until the cows come home, but if you don't fuel the fire, the fat's never going to burn," and they were right!

Every meal I eat includes protein, fat, and carbohydrates. Ninety percent of the time, I try to eat the highest quality food possible, but even when I eat a meal with lesser quality foods, I attempt to balance my plate. The simplest explanation of my method is that I eat a portion of protein equal to my portion of carbs. This will balance my blood sugar and then I add fat to slow digestion and keep me full.

I'm confident this works because many of my members recorded more than their food. My friend, who is a type-1 diabetic, routinely tracked her blood sugar. She knew unmatched carbohydrates caused her blood sugar to skyrocket, whereas balanced portions of protein and carbohydrates minimized the spike.

I also add water-rich vegetables to most meals and try to get a minimum of thirty servings weekly. Generally speaking, these are low-glycemic vegetables that soften when you cook them, and they are my go-to for seconds if I'm still hungry after a meal. I feel safe eating more lettuce, broccoli, or mushrooms because whoever gained weight by eating more veggies? They are also natural sources of critical vitamins, minerals, and antioxidants. Please note corn, peas, potatoes, or dried beans would not count as water-based; they have a place in a healthy meal but shouldn't be considered unlimited.

For breakfast, I often eat rice (Carbs) with quickly sauteed vegetables and an over-easy egg (Fat & Protein) or oatmeal (C) with peanut butter (F) and a low-sugar protein shake (P). I use half the recommended water when making the shake and pour it over my oats like cream. It's so, so yummy!

My snack might be a slice of pork loin (P and F) and an apple (C) or a few ounces of turkey breast,(P) a handful of grapes(C), and a handful of almonds (F).

Lunch and Dinner often consist of lean meat (P), a salad with sliced avocado (F), and a baked sweet potato (C).

So, what if I want a bowl of pasta? I add a protein like meatballs with marinara or grilled chicken breast with pesto. If I want pizza, I make (or order) one with protein (sausage, hamburger, or chicken) and lots of veggies, and I eat a salad on the side to help me avoid eating more slices than I want. Pizza is one of those things that tastes delicious today but will often make me feel crummy tomorrow.

What if you don't eat meat? You can still balance your meals. Soy is also a complete protein source, providing all essential amino acids, much like animal sources.

Many studies have suggested that increasing the consumption of plant foods like edamame and other soy products decreases the risk of obesity and overall mortality, diabetes, and heart disease and promotes a healthy complexion and hair, increased energy, and overall lower weight.

As with any food, it is better to consume tofu and other soy foods that have undergone minimal amounts of processing. I recommend avoiding convenience foods made with soy, such as meat and cheese substitutes.

Portion control is also important! When you sit down to eat, remember that you want to satisfy your hunger/energy needs- no more, no less. Of course, you want to enjoy your food, but you should also be aware of how much you eat. Learning to stop slightly before you feel satisfied is key to manageable weight loss. You should never feel "really hungry" before you eat or "really full" after you eat.

One trick is to take time to enjoy your food. Take a bite, set your fork down, and chew. Or talk with your dinner companions. Eat leisurely while sharing stories about the day. It's amazing how you can notice when you feel full when you try to let your stomach keep up with your mouth. Just because you can eat fast doesn't mean you should!

Another tip is to fill your plate in the kitchen before you sit down, leaving the extra food off the table. This simple act of out of sight-out of mind often allows me time to process my hunger cues without automatically grabbing an extra portion.

A food scale is another way to track your portions, but I feel like I'm "on a diet" when I'm weighing every morsel, so I've adopted the eyeball method of portioning using the guide below:

Protein- 1 serving = palm of a hand

Carbohydrate- (grains, starchy vegetables, and fruits)- 1 serving = 1 fist

Healthy fat- 1 serving = 1 thumb or a small handful of nuts

Water-based veggies - 1 serving = 2 hands cupped or more if you need

* Remember, if you're plating for your family, consider their portion equal to their hand, not yours. My husband and teenage boys frequently needed more food than I did.

Water is the final thing I've tried to incorporate into my daily routine. There have been times when the only water to cross my lips was carried on my toothbrush! Now, I try to drink eighty to one hundred ounces a day. This amount, I've learned, quenches my thirst and doesn't wake me up all night long. Keep track of your water in your food journal to find the perfect amount for you.

Drink water, sips at a time, all day long to avoid bathroom disruption. If you're new to drinking water, it might seem like you're making more trips to the restroom, but the urge will ease up after a couple of weeks as your body gets used to it.

I like to drink twelve to sixteen ounces of water first thing in the morning. Try hot water with lemon as a delicious alternative to coffee some mornings. I also like to add fruit and herbs to enhance the taste. Two of my favorite combinations are lemon and thyme or strawberry and basil. Ice water is great in the summer, but I find it easier to consume cool or room-temperature water during the colder months.

For all practical purposes, water is water. It is a part of every cell, tissue, organ, and body process. It helps regulate your body temperature, removes wastes, and carries nutrients, oxygen, and glucose to cells to give you energy. Water makes up sixty-five to seventy percent of your muscle tissue and keeps your body functioning efficiently.

Don't cheat yourself of its benefits by substituting soda, coffee, sugared/flavored water, sports drinks, fruit juices, etc. Reach your desired water goal, and then have something fun as a treat!

Wading In: Think about a food you love that makes you feel crummy. How can you enjoy it but limit your portion?

Deep Dive: Check the boxes. How varied is your diet? No judgement, just looking for opportunities!

Protein	☐ ☐ ☐ ☐ ☐ ☐ ☐ ☐ ☐
Fat	☐ ☐ ☐ ☐ ☐ ☐ ☐ ☐ ☐
Carbohydrates	☐ ☐ ☐ ☐ ☐ ☐ ☐ ☐ ☐
Vegetables	☐ ☐ ☐ ☐ ☐ ☐ ☐ ☐ ☐
Water	☐ ☐ ☐ ☐ ☐ ☐ ☐ ☐ ☐
Other Drinks	☐ ☐ ☐ ☐ ☐ ☐ ☐ ☐ ☐

♥

"Planning Vs. Prepping"

Are you a planner or a prepper?

I have friends who plan their meals each week and go to the grocery store to buy exactly what they need, and that works for them. I don't like to plan. It seems like I've written 15,000 weekly meal plans, and I think I've used two. This is often because of schedule changes or because I simply don't feel like eating what I planned to eat on the night I planned to eat it.

My weekly schedule is much more flexible now than when I had a full-time job and was trying to keep up with my guys. But freedom is not always a good thing. I'm often busy writing or sorting through a lifetime's worth of stuff and not paying attention to the time. Jeff is half a house away, stuck on his computer for work. We "forget" to eat throughout the day, and I know the first question he will ask me when he climbs up the stairs at 5:30 pm is, "What's for dinner?" When I planned, I would tell him, he would scrunch up his nose, and I would get mad.

This is not the way I want to spend my night.

One of my earliest members had a schedule that made mine look like I lived a life of leisure! Heather and her husband have two sets of twins spaced seven years apart, and they both work full-time jobs. She joined my first challenge, bringing co-workers, friends, and a sunny outlook from day one!

Jon followed her to the gym during the second session. They worked out together almost every day they were members. He would egg her on, and she'd raise a brow or crack a smile. She'd cheer him on, and he would work harder. They constantly amazed me with their ability to work together. They made life and love look easy.

We occasionally offered challenges at the gym for maintenance members; Heather and Jon would often participate. She was great at planning, and he was great at prepping (skills undoubtedly well rehearsed in their careers as a business office director and a chef). They attempted to teach their children to eat balanced along the way and shared a great idea. Heather separated snacks for the kids into bins labeled appropriately with Protein, Fat, and Carbs. The kids could choose from each one, guaranteeing them balance and variety. It would be great if everyone taught their kids to eat that way.

Heck, they did so well during their challenges, I figured out it was easier for my family to eat that way, and I abandoned my quest to be a planner and became a prepper.

Even now, with our nest empty, I still have containers of vegetables and fruit, cooked grains, hardboiled eggs, one or two kinds of meat, and a million ways to combine the ready-to-eat ingredients to keep us on track.

I know this method isn't going to work for everyone. Just yesterday, I talked to a friend who told me there was a time when decision fatigue was so great she would have probably looked in my fridge, felt overwhelmed, and decided to have toast or a couple of bowls of cereal for dinner! If you are a repetitive eater and like to know what you will have, by all means, continue that!

This method of prepping has helped me save money. Cleaning the fridge used to be a once-a-month thing for me. Now that fewer people are eating here, the little jars and bowls of leftovers get lost much easier than the large containers did. This task has bumped up the priority list to a weekly chore. I sort through leftovers and decide what to eat immediately, what to freeze, and what to toss. I also go through my produce drawer to see what needs to be used up before I go to the store and purchase more.

Confession: I collect fruits and veggies like some women collect shoes, and I've been known to forget the most perfect little eggplant in the bottom of the drawer until it is unrecognizable.

My new "clean the fridge first" system has helped me cut waste considerably. I pull the still edible (but sad and limp) veggies out to make stock and place the "good" ones in a large plastic container to be used first. If something is questionable and has the potential to ruin the flavor of a dish, I toss it. Most importantly. I check things off my grocery list so I don't buy something I already have.

Usually, after cleaning the fridge, I make breakfast, trying to use leftover meat and veggies in a hash or quiche.

I rinse the dishes and start the dishwasher so everything is ready when I get home to prep.

Grocery shopping used to be a hit-or-miss thing. I'd fly in after work, grab something that sounded good, and arrive home to discover I already had half of the items I purchased in the cupboard or I completely forgot the one thing I really needed to make a specific dish. Now, I like to shop before the rest of the world wakes up so I can wander the aisles and pick just the right things. My list might include specifics like olive oil, Parmesan, or oats, but it also lists some general items like "vegetables and fruit." I don't buy food if it doesn't look good or smell fresh, so I don't usually put specific produce items on the list.

I peruse the whole produce section first, checking quality and price. Often, you'll find great buys in the organic section, but if you've already picked up what you want in the front of the store, you won't take time to look.

If I'm buying greens, I buy tubs that have been washed and prepped. I eat more salad if it's ready to go and fits better in my fridge.

When buying vegetables, I always look for firm, bright colors and no sign of decay.

If I buy fruit, I look for bright colors, then raise it towards me, inhaling deeply. If it smells "like fruit," I'll inspect further and look for signs of decay. Why smell? Due to high off-season demand, some foods are grown and ripened in environments that don't allow the flavors to come through. For example, yesterday, I saw some beautiful, bright strawberries. I picked up the box to smell them, but there was no smell. Nothing. How do you think they are going to taste? Exactly! Like nothing. I'd rather buy frozen than settle for something marginal that will spoil in my fridge.

When I get home, I unload the dishwasher and fill the sink with hot, soapy water so I can clean as I go. I boil two pots of water on the stove, one for oats or rice and another for veggie scraps that will become stock, and start hardboiled eggs in the pressure cooker. I unpack my groceries, placing ready-to-go items (yogurt, milk, berries, etc.) in the fridge, leaving everything I'll need for prep time on the counter.

Meal Prep will consume the next hour or so. It's a small price to pay, considering the time it saves me in the week ahead.

I start vegetable prep first. If I'm making something in the slow cooker for dinner that night, I'll place the insert on the counter to add as I go. The scraps, like green onion tops, pepper innards, celery centers, etc., immediately go into the pot of water on the stove to simmer while I work.

- Raw peppers, celery, cauliflower, grape tomatoes, pea pods, and radishes get washed first, cut, and then arranged in a large plastic container lined with dry white paper towels.
- Next, I clean hearty fruits, like grapes, place them in a paper towel-lined container, and make fruit ice cubes with lemons and berries.
- I finish adding ingredients to the slow cooker and make marinades for meat if that's in the plan.
- Finally, I cut onions if I need them for recipes, so the flavor doesn't carry through everything else.

- I place cooked oats in individual containers after it cools.
- I toss the rice in a colander, rinse it with cool water, and toss it a few times to get as much water as possible off. Then, I spread it on a large baking sheet lined with parchment paper and pop it in the freezer for an hour or two. The individual grains freeze, and you can store the rice in a large freezer bag, scooping out only what you need for a particular meal. It heats up quickly on the stove with a bit of broth or water!

*This freeze method also works great for fresh berries or fruit slices.

- The hardboiled eggs go into ice water, allowing them to cool completely before storing them in the fridge. I like to peel the eggs and keep them in a large glass jar with a lid so the smell doesn't impact the rest of the food throughout the week.
- If I cook beans for the week, I cool them too and store them in glass jars with some of the cooking liquid. I've included an easy pressure cooker recipe in the Back of the Book.

As much as I hope this helps, I know it doesn't cover it all. You're likely sitting there thinking, "Great… I have a bunch of stuff cut up, but now what?".

I use all of this prepped food for snacks or as quick ingredients for other recipes I might make during the week. This routine has made it easier for me to eat healthy (and stress less). There are several recipes and examples of repurposing ingredients in the appendix!

We have a large chest freezer in our garage and have purchased half a beef and a whole hog for several years. It's a significant investment once a year, but considering the average cost per pound is a fraction of the grocery store price, I highly recommend it if you can swing it. I also buy oversized packages of chicken, divide them into several one-recipe portions, and freeze them. If you watch for sales, you can save a lot of money.

After I finish prep, I look through the freezer and pull two or three packages of meat to the fridge to thaw. I try to cook one large amount of protein to stretch over a couple of meals, but I repurpose it so it doesn't feel like we're always eating leftovers.

Pork Roast on Wednesday might become carnitas on Friday. A whole roasted chicken (or two) could be eaten for dinner on Sunday, the leftover meat can be turned into chicken salad for sandwiches, and the carcass can be used to make broth for soup. Black beans cooked in the pressure cooker can be used on a salad or made into a soup or dip for fresh vegetables. Taco meat cooked for dinner tonight can be mixed in with scrambled eggs for breakfast or turned into nachos on game day.

Remember, I may not necessarily have a plan, but when I have fresh foods available, I will always win.

Wading In: Are you a prepper or a planner?

Deep Dive: What could you cook this week to repurpose into another meal?

♥

Crowding Out in the Kitchen

Crowding out might be the single best "tool" to use when making changes to your diet. It's a gentle, progressive way to eat and drink better. It's not complicated, and it won't ever make you feel like you're missing out.

Most of us know which foods we should reserve as treats, but if you're my age, there's a chance that you have been eating sugar-sweetened and flavor-enhanced foods and artificially sweetened drinks your whole life. Ours was the first generation to be exposed to cream-filled, chocolatey treats sealed in cellophane, pasta in a can, or juice in a box. Our taste buds and our dopamine receptors have been trained to expect more than real food can deliver. Broccoli rarely triggers moments of ecstasy like a bowl of chocolate chip cookie dough ice cream can.

So what's a girl to do when she decides to eat more whole foods and doesn't want to suffer from cravings, headaches, and withdrawal?

I threw out a poll on Instagram, asking my followers what they generally gave up when they were trying to "get healthy" and the bane of their diet plan- the food and drinks that routinely tripped them up.

Most people gave up bread, sugar, and alcohol when they started a diet, and many shared that they fell back to their old ways for pizza, pasta, chocolate, and wine.

I've had several members who had daily habits when they joined the gym. I encountered the most memorable one early in my career. This woman had everything going for her. She was smart, had a great attitude, support at home, and a desire to change. The problem was she consumed several glasses of highly caffeinated citrus soda every day.

There were two significant barriers in the way. She was never going to reach her goals, given the amount of liquid sugar she consumed, and would have suffered painful consequences if she quit cold turkey. There was simply no way to go to zero without feeling terrible. Headaches and other withdrawal symptoms can cause a person to "break" and consume the offending substance. The moment the pain subsides, the wicked witch of shame shows up, and suddenly, change is beyond reach again.

My suggestion was a taper (a.k.a. crowding out). I asked her to start by becoming aware of how many portions she drank in a day. After confirming her routine, I asked her to remove the one that meant the least (you know, the one you drink without tasting because you're busy doing something else). I suggested she drink a glass of water with a heavy squeeze of lemon. After a couple of days, she took out the next least important. She slowly crowded out, so her dopamine receptors didn't even realize what was happening! Her replacement didn't have to be water. Ice tea, flavored water, or sparkling water worked too. Over time, her "need" for the highly caffeinated citrus soda turned into a choice once in a while!

You can use the crowding out method for more than soda! Check out my suggestions for the top diet disruptors below:

- **Coffee**: Do you think you can't function without a pot of coffee? Make ¾ pot tomorrow… ½ pot next week. A cup next month. Take the time to enjoy it while it's hot rather than letting it sit around- you might actually drink less than you think.
- **Highly sweetened coffee creamer**: Crowd out by measuring. If you use four tablespoons on day one (you'll be surprised

how much it takes to make it the color you're used to), cut back to three tomorrow and substitute your milk of choice for the last tablespoon. Keep reducing slowly over the next several weeks until you break your habit and treat yourself to an unsweetened latte from your favorite coffee shop to celebrate.

- **Ice cream**: Do you remember when ice cream was a reward for cleaning your plate? What was undoubtedly intended as an incentive has often been cited as the start of many sweet tooth habits. Ice cream is a treat many of us enjoy, but people usually try to work it in by buying fat-free, sugar-free frozen ice-like products that leave them unsatisfied and wanting more. I suggest picking a night each week and eating the best ice cream money can buy. Measure out a portion and eat it slowly, savoring every bite. If you can't resist it calling to you from the freezer mid-week, plan a memorable trip to an ice cream shop and enjoy it somewhere beautiful, like a park.
- **Salty snacks**: Ditch the chips!! Popcorn popped in flavored oil is one of my favorite treats. Also, nuts or a few whole-grain pretzels. If you want to buy chips for an event or because your turkey sandwich isn't the same without a handful on the side, buy a snack-size bag so they are used up quickly.
- **Chocolate**: Okay ladies. Many of you shared that you deserve chocolate once a month (all week long). And I agree. But purchase the best chocolate you can afford. Break it up into daily portions and eat it only when the world is quiet, the TV is off, and you have the presence of mind to fully enjoy how incredible it makes you feel. A shareable size bag of candy-coated discs is not worthy of your attention! Get what you deserve! Rest the chocolate on your tongue and let it begin to melt. Savor it slowly.
- **Fast food:** Learn to cook with planned leftovers. Grilled sirloin for dinner tonight can be fajitas on Thursday. Roasted chicken on Sunday can become chicken salad sandwiches to take to work. If you need a meal to go, wrap your protein in a tortilla and head on out the door! It can help you trim your waistline and save you a significant amount of money.

- **Snack food**: Don't eat vegetables? Or worse, you hate vegetables? Reconsider how you eat them: salsa, breakfast bowls (cauliflower rice), roasted veggies as a thickener in sauces, or blended into spaghetti sauce. Or eat them with a dip; my three favorites are peanut butter mixed 1:1 with Greek yogurt, hummus, or black bean. All three recipes are included in the Back of the Book!
- **Pizza**: Make your own! Try the crustless recipe in the back or order delivery and eat a salad before you dive in!
- **Wine**: Ha! I feel this one personally. If I were answering those Instagram questions, my answer to both would have been wine. I knew I had to change my daily wine habit to lose weight and improve my health, so I started experimenting with shrubs, juices, and sparkling waters to cut the calories and still enjoy an adult-tasting drink at the end of the day.

♥

Deep Dive: Food Journal

As I've tried to emphasize throughout this chapter, there isn't a perfect diet, but there is a perfect diet for you. Unfortunately, you didn't come with an instruction manual, so you will have to figure this out on your own.

I feel best when I eat a diet balanced with proteins, fats, carbohydrates, and vegetables daily, and I stay engaged and excited about mealtime when I eat different foods every day. I know which foods cause heartburn and which give me gas. I've figured out breakfast combinations that keep me satisfied all morning, and I know which comfort foods will leave me hungry within an hour or two.

You can have this knowledge, too, if you take the time to record your food and drink for a while. I recommend at least three months to get a good feel for the foods that make you thrive and those that make you feel less than ideal. You don't need to worry about tracking portion sizes or calories- just eat, write, and record how you feel.

I shared two different styles of journals in the back of the book. Both have worked for me at different times and for different reasons. The written style helped me identify foods that aggravate my auto-immune symptoms. The bullet style is good to help me keep track if I'm tired or just feeling "off." Sometimes, I forget to eat, which means I'm also low on veggies and water! I hope you find one that works for you!

You can download a copy of the bullet point journal at kimmosimanwellness.com/journal

Chapter 6

Your Calling

Refocus

For the first fifty-five years of my life, I've been a do-er, a pleaser, often a loner, and perhaps an over-achiever. It's common for me to set my plans aside to help someone else accomplish theirs, even if it means long hours working alone. Sometimes, if the project is big enough, like a wedding, I'd let it consume me (sorry kids!). Most of the time, I enjoy helping because, deep down, all I've ever wanted to do is love people and do a few extra little things to bring more joy to their world. Helping makes me happy, even when I over-commit. There have been moments when I felt over my head, but nothing is better than the feeling of a job well done.

As I'm settling into this new, slower life and learning to appreciate everyday moments more often, I've come to realize how overbearing I must have been at times. I wasn't striving for perfection, but I'm sure from the outside, it looked like that was my only goal.

As a child and a young adult (heck, who am I kidding? It still happens on occasion), there were many moments when I thought I had to prove myself worthy of love. There never seemed to be enough A+ on the report card or personal bests in the pool- so I pushed myself towards perfection. I pushed and pushed until I cracked and broke all the rules in high school. If I can't be good enough, I might as well be bad, right?

As I moved into adulthood, I still strived for perfection. My mantra seemed to be, "Let me convince you to love me by doing all the things that *really* don't matter to you." People-pleasing, high-achieving, hard-working Kim got burnt out and hurt again and again because I couldn't seem to let go of *doing* long enough to BE with another person.

As a wife, I tried to do it all: work my outside job, clean, cook, manage the schedules, handle the bills, and be a gracious host. I set my role in stone by not communicating effectively for many years. I didn't ask for help when I felt overwhelmed but retaliated by huffing, puffing, and falling asleep on the couch to avoid a fight. Didn't he know when I needed help? Couldn't he see that I was tired? Hmm… shouldn't I know he couldn't read my mind?

As a parent, I called myself engaged and helpful. Looking back, it's more likely I tried to play the role of super mom because I was afraid I wouldn't be good enough for the boys to love me once they had a choice. I tried to earn their love by creating the most wonderful experiences and opportunities. If I helped them with their homework, remained lenient with the curfews, and threw the perfect graduation party, wasn't it guaranteed they would love me forever?

I did the same thing with work at the gym. I was always available and tried to accommodate every wish, answering emails into the wee hours and bending payment plans so members would stay forever! No one could teach like I could, and no one else would stay for hours after class just to listen. I wanted everyone to know I would do whatever I had to for them to succeed.

Once upon a time, I believed if I could make someone's life better, they would love me forever. I also thought, through my giving, that person should know that's how I loved and would automatically give me what I needed in return. Now, I know (and my people know) that I show love through acts of service, even if they don't. I've tried to learn to use my words to reinforce my feelings and communicate what I need to feel appreciated and loved.

I've also realized that no one in my life expects me to be perfect, whether personal or professional. No one will love me less or unfriend me if I'm not the best. My husband loves me when I'm crabby and discouraged or feeling gross, and he helps me with chores, even when he knows I'll redo what he did. My sons and daughters-in-law love me through my senior moments, recipe failures, and ridiculous gifts. I've learned to join in once in a while when they enjoy a good laugh at my expense! I have family and friends who love me unconditionally, whether we see each other occasionally or once a week, even if I forget a special date or if I'm running late.

And even though I will never be perfect on this side of heaven, I am loved by a God who thinks I'm lovely just as I am. He offers me grace when I goof up and the excellent gift of knowing I am loved no matter what I do, look like, say, or feel.

"But by the grace of God, I am what I am, and His grace to me was not without effect."

1 Corinthians 15:10

I read those words today, and somehow, through the rush of catching up on my weekly passages, they stood out. I reread them, accepting them as if they were written just for me. I reached for another version just to be sure I understood. The Message worded it this way:

"But because God was so gracious, so very generous, here I am..."

I am imperfect but wonderfully made.

I am forgetful, but I remember what is special about you.

I am often late, but I'll make time for you.

I bite off more than I can chew, but I want you to feel special.

I'm easily bored, but I am passionate about things that matter.

I am right even when I'm wrong, but I know how to say I'm sorry.

"...and I'm not about to let His grace go to waste":

I was created with gifts unique only to me.

I've been placed in this time and this place with my own set of stories.

My circumstances allow me to do His will and to be of service to others.

My busy days are gone, and now is the time to create opportunities for community.

I often stop myself, wondering if this is what I'm truly meant to do. Is it possible that all roads could lead to this moment in time? In my greatest moments of doubt, I've always received an answer that made me believe again.

But because God was so gracious… here I am.

Consider your unique gifts.

Wading In: How have you used them in the past?

Deep Dive: How can you refocus your efforts to serve others now?

Nudges

Life is a journey filled with unexpected encounters and experiences that shape us into who we become. These moments often lead us down uncharted paths and, in hindsight, appear destined to be part of our story.

Throughout my life, I've been keenly aware of my gut feelings, relying on them as a guiding force. As I attempt to give up a little control, I find myself experiencing moments where I feel nudged in a particular direction or placed in precisely the right spot at the right time. The frequency of these occurrences has left me with a lingering sense of wonder and makes me question whether it's me or the Spirit at play.

Gut feelings, also known as intuition, are those instinctive, visceral reactions we experience when facing decisions or situations. In the past, I would attempt to squash these feelings due to their irrational nature. As I've learned to trust, I've discovered my gut will rarely lead me astray.

Nudges are subtle, persistent feelings or thoughts that encourage us to make specific decisions or take certain actions. They often come when we least expect them and may gently push us to pursue new opportunities or make choices that align with our life's purpose. Over the last year, I've met some of the most incredible people because I sensed a need to sign up for a course or accept an invitation.

Serendipity refers to the occurrence of fortunate and unexpected events or discoveries by chance. It's those moments when we stumble upon something meaningful or meet someone who profoundly impacts our lives seemingly out of nowhere. While serendipity can be attributed to luck or random circumstances, I sense they are gifts- experiences or people put in place just for me.

Lately, I've opened my heart to the Holy Spirit as a source of inspiration, guidance, and comfort. I attribute my gut feelings, nudges, and serendipitous moments to the workings of the Spirit. I like to think of them as answered prayers guiding me toward a particular path or purpose. Doors open when I follow the Spirit's lead.

These gentle touches often manifest as subtle yet persistent feelings or thoughts, prompting me to step out of my comfort zone and embark on new adventures. One of the most remarkable aspects of nudges is their ability to lead us to people who can profoundly impact our lives. It's as if the Holy Spirit orchestrates encounters that align with our spiritual growth and personal development. These connections often occur at just the right time, and the individuals we meet become catalysts for transformative experiences.

You may feel prompted to volunteer for a charitable cause you've never considered before. Through this endeavor, you cross paths with like-minded individuals whose passion and dedication inspire you to make a more significant impact on the world.

Additionally, they can lead us toward personal growth and self-discovery. I often find myself nudged to explore new avenues, seek different perspectives, or pursue practices that help me better understand myself and the world around me. These transformative moments can provide clarity, personal development, and a deeper faith.

Recognizing and embracing these moments can be a profound aspect of your spiritual journey. They can lead us toward new experiences, transformative encounters, and personal growth. They remind us that divine guidance is available if we listen and follow. By doing so, we can open ourselves up to a world of possibilities, connections, and purpose that can profoundly impact not only our lives but the lives of others.

Wading In: How do you respond to nudges in your life?

Deep Dive: Have you ever shut the Spirit down?
How can you be open to opportunities in your life?

♥

Dream

"Every great dream begins with a dreamer. Always remember, you have within you the strength, the patience, and the passion to reach for the stars to change the world."

~ Harriet Tubman[1]

I approach the noise with a platter in my hands. There are twenty people or so gathered around one long table. There is candlelight and conversations, stories, and laughter. Jeff is sitting at the end. He looks up at me and smiles, and everyone at the table stops and turns to me as well, waiting with anticipation to see what I prepared for the feast. I don't know a single person, and somehow it's okay.

This is my recurring dream. Maybe it's a vision of Heaven, new friends gathered around a table, breaking bread, and sharing a simple meal. I have to be honest; I hope I'm not placed on kitchen duty once I pass through the pearly gates!

I think it's more likely a sign that I'm supposed to help bring people together- to find a common place for people to build relationships for companionship and support… to create a place of belonging, comfort, and love.

I think I did that when I ran the gym. Mardi and Sandy, the ladies who helped me get my start in the fitness world, created an environment that felt like family, and I strived to establish that same feeling when I opened my location. Working out in a group helps develop camaraderie amongst the members like nothing else because you're all going through the same torture together! Just kidding! Nothing is better than building friendships and establishing accountability while getting healthy. We also encouraged teamwork through partner exercises and peer-led coaching. I've met many of my forever friends through connections made at the gym.

Once I closed the business, I felt an incredible void in my life. People I had seen every day for years were suddenly gone. I'd catch myself thinking, 'I can't wait to share this recipe with Tammy or try a new kickboxing routine with Kori,' only to be disappointed that I wouldn't see them again soon.

There's something really good about sharing your life with other people. Whether it's family, friends, co-workers, Bible study members, or workout partners, the people in your circle often hold you accountable as you reach for your goals.

When I retired, I had no one to answer to except Jeff and myself. He loves me a little too much to keep me on task. I might not have loved myself enough. As my weight climbed, my insecurities did as well. I quit accepting invitations to go out. If he wanted to go, I'd cook a great meal and open a good bottle of wine to convince him we should stay home. If a friend would ask me to go for a walk, I'd often claim to be too busy. It's easier to pretend to be okay when you're in hiding.

Once COVID changed the social gathering rules and I couldn't spend time with my closest family and friends, I realized how much I missed it. My seclusion was no longer a choice but a necessity. I vowed to make community a priority again if we all made it through.

As I shared at the beginning of this chapter, I have a dream. I love to cook, be social (on my terms), and want to bring people together. But as great as my dream is, it doesn't have to be yours. Part of finding joy in the journey is learning to accept your gifts and allowing them to inspire your dreams. Life has incredible purpose when you're doing what you're meant to do, and it's even better when your purpose sets you down right in the middle of a new group of friends!

Several years ago, I had a friend whom I'd met through my gym. She was the best listener and observer I'll ever know. She would throw a question out into space through her blog or at a dinner party and then just listen. There were rarely follow-up questions, but sometimes, she'd ask another if she sensed the opportunity to go a little deeper.

Alison was quiet at the gym, often working out by herself. I got the sense she worked through work projects or ideas as she exercised, much as I do now on my walks. She may have been alone for an hour but often jumped into conversation after class. She engaged people, and she loved knowing what they thought. She frequently took notes and was eager to learn more about an opportunity or resource she discovered through conversation.

She was curious, always learning, and had a deep love for people, so it was no surprise when she and her husband decided to embark on a new-to-them, once-a-month tradition of *Spaghetti Saturdays*[2]. They would extend invitations throughout the month, set tables up all over their house, and prepare a big batch of pasta and sauce. There was music and candlelight and an always-changing group of individuals who would wander through their door. Such a lovely idea and so brave! They moved to a new city, but I often think of them and wonder if they have continued their tradition.

In the years since attending my last Spaghetti Saturday, I've longed to establish a repeating gathering of my own. Still, with my husband's work schedule, it's always been impossible to set a regular day and time that would stick.

I've considered weekly dinner parties, but as much as I love my current friends, I want to get to know new people, mix them in with the old, or maybe even be so brave as to fill my table with strangers. It might be fun to pass out invitations as I walk down the street, but it feels a little risky, and I hope to create something that could continue even when I'm away.

As the process takes shape, I envision a larger gathering than I can host at home, so I'm working through a plan, and I hope to implement it at church! It seems safer than passing out random invitations. I could fill a table with "strangers" who belong to an existing community and ask them to join me in sharing the love.

Since this is my dream, I feel like I'm allowed to create the rules! I would extend twenty invitations to random people, not friend groups or book clubs. As loving as each member might be, most groups still feel exclusive to those who don't belong. My mission is to bring people together without making them feel like they're still "on the outside."

Maybe a large dinner party isn't your thing. I've talked to several people who shudder at the thought of cooking for twenty. What if you made the group smaller and cooked burgers in the backyard?

I started following the business *Neighbor's Table*[3] on Instagram. They build large picnic tables and benches to deliver all over the country to bring people together! The best part of their organization is that the delivery team joins the table's new owners for a meal on delivery day. How wonderful to bring strangers together with the hope of building a world of friends!

Is that idea still too big? Could you invite someone to join you for coffee? Or ask a neighbor to gather around the fire pit for s'mores?

Candles lit, conversation cards in place, or coffee in a paper cup; the blessing of new friends breaking bread, and love are well worth the effort. If you're ever in town, look me up! I'd love to share a meal with you.

Wading In: How could you share a meal with someone this week?

Deep Dive: Extend the invitation!

♥

Simple Gatherings

Community is crucial for personal growth as it offers a sense of belonging, support, and inspiration in different areas of life, including spirituality and education. Being part of a group with shared beliefs and experiences allows for mutual support, which can be especially helpful during tough times and in staying committed to goals. Encouragement from like-minded individuals reinforces our beliefs and journey.

I've shared over and over again that I like to host meals in my home. It's my thing- it doesn't have to be yours. What do you like to do? If cooking for other people seems unimaginable, start a book club. Create a walking group if you don't want to bring people into your home. Host a knitting club at a coffee shop.

It's easy! Identify something that interests you, pick a place, invite a close friend or two, and ask them to bring a friend. Or reach out to those peripheral friends, you know, the ones who say "Hi" at work or smile at you in church (but you don't know a thing about them). Voila! You have the beginnings of a community!

Several years back, when the gym was still open, I had a different book forming in my mind, and I thought it might be helpful to gather some women together to see if the idea would take hold or flush itself out.

I invited several gym members to dinner and then slipped into panic mode:

What would I serve?

How was I going to get the house clean?

Where can I find matching dishes?

Could I get the bathroom remodeled in time?!?

One morning, a few days before my guests would arrive, I was sitting at the breakfast table, making yet another list. I must have been talking to myself because out of nowhere, my husband said, "Knowing the group you invited, there will be so much conversation around the table, no one will notice the house's condition unless you bring it up. And soup is good."

These are wise words, and I try to remember them whenever we host in our home.

I made soup, salad, and dessert. I bought bread. I lit candles and pulled out my grandma's dishes (The everyday ones… they aren't fancy, but still special because they are pretty and they match). I made a gallon of flavored water and sat down to plan our discussion.

I invited these friends to join me to discuss the idea of balance and how it fits into maintaining a healthy life. This first meeting was detail-oriented as I hoped to convey my vision and schedule future meetings. I was surprised when most of the participants were able to commit to meetings during the holiday season and encouraged by their willingness to share.

Unlike the classes I taught in the gym, I wasn't trained for this discussion. My book idea stemmed from a deep-down hunch that most of us are the same. I believe that women, in general, want to make permanent lifestyle changes, but because of the give and take that exists in everyday life, they can't seem to balance their desire to be thin and healthy, profitable and loving, spiritual and happy all at the same time!

The proof came over dinner, surrounded by this group of women. We came together to tear apart my theory and build something worthwhile and true- to create something that could enrich our lives and be shared with others. I couldn't have been more pleased with the discussions and the promise of something really good, but that night, our meeting was so much more than a project- it was exactly what I needed.

These women (whom I knew but didn't know one another) opened up and started talking. The book could have been written that night if I had taken notes, but I got so wrapped up in the conversation that I forgot to grab my journal. I could have listened to them for hours. They used words like discipline, manage, and escape. They finished each other's sentences. There was so much wisdom, grace, and strength sitting around my dining room table: strong, capable women who have "checked off" many of life's daunting tasks. And yet, through the storytelling, it became clear that we all had times when we felt we weren't "enough."

I wrapped things up near the end of the meal, with an assignment to identify what was "enough" and to try to exceed those expectations every day during the coming week.

Imagine the power of lying your head on your pillow each night and saying, "Today was a good day," rather than "Tomorrow, I'll do better."

As I sit here reminiscing, I long to expand this slower life. I want to create situations where I can spend hours learning and sharing with those who will carve out time for me. A life in which I spend my time focusing on self-awareness rather than self-improvement.

Perhaps I have discovered an opportunity to enrich this life I love. Invite a few friends, ask a good question, and enjoy the goodness of soup.

Wading In: How was today a good day?
Who did you share it with?

Deep Dive: What pulls you out of balance?
Is there something you could change?

Family First

I love the holidays, especially Thanksgiving. It's a love that started with my grandparents when I was a little girl and has been fostered by my mom throughout my life.

When I was a child, all the businesses closed, so it didn't matter what was happening in our lives, we were free to celebrate together. We didn't have cell phones and iPads to distract us. Cable TV and VCRs didn't exist, so we couldn't escape the day with Hallmark movie marathons. And stores didn't open at 4:00 pm- in fact, they didn't open until the next day!

Thanksgiving was a day for family and friends. In my earliest memories, I'd wake up and wander to the kitchen. Mom would be there making a cake or a pie to take to my grandparents. She always had some sweet treats and cocoa for Shelley and me to eat while we waited for the Macy's parade to begin.

Later in the day, we'd travel across town to Grandma and Grandpa's house. The moment we arrived, it "felt like Thanksgiving". There was always a big hug for Kimmie just inside the front door. The house was warm and noisy, and it smelled like heaven. I'm not sure if it was the turkey or the 50 other dishes that magically appeared from the oven that created the smell, but it always made me happy.

The best years were those when my cousins came to dinner. There were six of us, all girls, within years of each other, and we always got to sit together at a table in the kitchen that Grandma set just for us. The best thing about the "girls' table" was that we could eat and talk about anything. No adult eyes on us!

Our Christmas celebration was equally special but different. We would go to my grandparent's house on Christmas Eve. You could see their house from a block away. It was lit up with multi-colored lights, plastic Santa and his reindeer on the roof, and the shimmering silver tree glowing in changing technicolor through the window.

Christmas was casual and festive. The little house was packed with three generations of family, the adults sipping on Pink Squirrels or Grasshoppers in the kitchen and all of us little girls dancing to the lights that pulsed on the front of Grandpa's bar while the built-in 8-track player blasted holiday favorites. We'd laugh, play, and run off to the kitchen to beg for Shirley Temples when we'd had enough fun.

I've celebrated more than one hundred of those special days, receiving thousands of gifts and eating mountains of homemade treats, but the memories that linger closest to my heart are those with family. The whole family. Grandma and Grandpa's siblings and their kids, my aunts and uncles and cousins, his, hers and whoever's. And it makes me sad that we no longer make time for that.

Holidays were always a big production, but as my generation grew up, married, and had kids, getting everyone together became harder and harder. Someone always had a tournament to go to or a deer tag to fill. Others had to go over the river or through the woods to another grandma's house.

It seems that in a world where we've been given time-saving technology, everyone should be able to set aside at least one day a year to gather with the people they love.

I miss the extended family gatherings, but I also miss the regular nightly dinner ritual at the table when my boys were growing up. No matter how busy we were, it seemed we could reconnect as a family when we shared a meal at the end of the day.

I know many families who divide and conquer with activities after school, eating meals from a paper bag in the car as they run from one place to another. I was hopeful that more people would discover the value of family meals when we were forced to stay in during the pandemic. I hoped we would learn to appreciate a life of "less is more." But on the back side of COVID-19, we, as a society, seem to be busier than ever.

I'm an efficient cook. After thirty years working in restaurants, it would be pretty disappointing if I wasn't. I run my kitchen at home the same way I would have prepared for lunch rush back in the day, and as much as I welcome people to my kitchen, I don't want any help. I always have a plan and like things done in a certain way- if you've ever cooked with me, I'm sure you'll agree (and please know I'm sorry if I've ever shooed you away)!

There are two exceptions to my no-help rule, and I gave birth to both! I'm convinced my sons are good cooks because I taught them most of what I know, but I'm sure they'd tell you it was despite it! (I kept a few secrets, so I'll always have an edge!)

When they were in middle school, we started a fun little weekly tradition called Boy's Night. They'd work to plan a meal, I'd shop when they were at school, and they'd cook for the family. The meals were usually basic, but Boy's Night gave them experience in the kitchen (and, selfishly, time with me.)

I came up with this idea for a couple of reasons. It taught them an important skill that will benefit them throughout their lives. As they became comfortable in the kitchen, they could prepare healthy meals and delicious food instead of relying solely on processed or takeout food.

As they researched recipes and selected ingredients for their meals, we had the opportunity to learn about balance, and they often included a variety of fruits, vegetables, whole grains, and lean proteins in their meals. It was fun to watch them attempt to include ingredients we hadn't tried before!

It also instilled a sense of creativity in both boys. Zachary was picky when he was younger but is an adventurous cook now. He likes to explore new methods and has become quite accomplished in baking and sous vide cooking. Samuel loves to try different cuisines and has developed a love of spice- I still catch him in MY kitchen adding to the pot to make my meals "better." He used to talk about opening a restaurant- who knows, maybe someday!

One of my favorite memories is the Christmas Challenge we dreamed up a few years ago. It was like Boy's Night but with a new set of rules!

The boys and their wives arrived the night before our formal family meal to eat, drink, and play cards. Little did they know they would be cooking that night. We separated the couples and had them answer family trivia questions to earn chances to procure pre-purchased food items for their culinary creations. There were cans of meat, uncommon vegetables, and various strange-flavored condiments. Jeff and I were advisors but "hands off" for the competition. Watching them brainstorm and bump and slide through the kitchen was fun. We laughed until we cried, sampled mostly edible food, and then enjoyed pizza delivery!

Cooking and sharing a meal is one of my favorite things. Boys Night was a reason for all of us to be home, around the table together. It was a mountainous task some weeks, but we did it. Although they're grown now, we still try to find a way to cook together and share a meal as often as possible.

I tried to get Zach to give up his famous Mac & Cheese recipe, but he's still keeping it a secret- maybe I'll convince him by the next book!

It's a never-ending challenge to see if I can keep some of the traditions from my childhood alive. We don't have grand celebrations like my grandparents, but we try to stay in touch with those we love. I'd love the opportunity to create that special holiday feeling I remember so well. Last November, as I pulled out my favorite recipes from years past, it occurred to me- that it's never been about the bird, the gravy, or even the pie; the heart of the meal has always been how I felt.

Memories of hugs from my grandparents, giggles with my cousins, my parent's laughter, and love from my husband and children are what I remember most fondly- not the food or the gifts. Heck, I don't even care if we celebrate on the actual holiday. Any day is okay if I am surrounded by the people I love.

Think about your childhood.

Wading In: What is your favorite holiday memory?

Deep Dive: How have your memories inspired your current traditions?

♥

Inspiration

"Don't let anyone look down on you because you are young, but set an example for the believers in speech, in conduct, in love, in faith, and in purity."

1 Timothy 4:12

We were handed a card as we entered the auditorium that Sunday morning and told to wait for instructions. I sat in my seat, situated my bag, and looked at the paper in my hand- it was a prayer card. My heart started to pick up the pace. I don't like interactive church, and I don't like to share (at least not face-to-face!). I like to keep my prayers between God and myself, plus everything is going well right now… what do I need someone to pray for?

The music started, and I was transported to a familiar place of comfort and worship. The second song started to close, and the worship leader began to pray. Lost in the words, I couldn't tell you what she said, but she closed with a call to put our prayer requests on the paper we'd been handed. They could be anonymous. We could share our burdens and joys, knowing someone would pray for us later that night.

I stared at the card… I didn't have to fill it out. No one would know. Hundreds of others were in the church- no one would miss mine. My dear friends sat next to me, scribbling away. "I wonder what they're worried about," I thought as I lifted my head to plead with God to forgive me for my non-participation. I noticed the rows of students in front of me. The college year had just begun, and the front pews were packed.

Young men and women sat in their chairs, heads down, writing frantically to fill the card. I'll never know the words on those cards, but the emotion that surged in me was unmistakable, and the nudge to dig deep was obvious.

It occurs to me that these young people taught me an important lesson: Faith is different for everyone, and trends have changed throughout history. While my generation might have relied on memorization, hymnal worship, and Sunday school lessons to introduce us to God, young people today seem to prefer to experience God rather than simply know about Him.

We were taught you don't talk about religion or politics. Fortunately, that time has passed, and more and more people feel comfortable sharing their beliefs. I'm sure it's easier with social media, but even now, I find myself standing in awe at the profound expression of faith through prayer, song, or even a posture in church and online.

I prayed that morning for faith like theirs. Faith that would allow me to bear myself, to release my worry and joy, and to trust in the prayers of strangers and the goodness of my God.

A few days later, I volunteered to help set up a large worship service in the center of our college campus. As I arrived, I was struck by how many young people took time out of their busy school day to help. While assembling a tent, I had the good fortune to meet several more college students and a recent graduate who coordinated the campus worship. I shared how much I was touched by the students on Sunday morning and asked if there was a way I could thank them for their display of unwavering faith.

Through a series of emails and organization, I was able to cook for the twenty young men and women who volunteered their time to lead other college students on their journey. I love that I can provide the opportunity for a home-cooked meal and a time for fellowship.

Over the last year, I participated in a couple of mixed-generational classes at church, and again, I'm amazed at the students' willingness to share and give their time. Stories are swapped between us, and there seems to be a quiet acceptance of one another's experiences. I haven't witnessed any moments of "that's the old way" but instead many instances of "tell me more." In all truth, I'm a little jealous. If my faith had been nurtured as much as theirs in my twenties, I can only imagine the comfort it would have brought me through many of life's trials.

Many of these young people volunteer at church, in our community, and worldwide through mission trips. I'm amazed at their bravery and their willingness to serve. My niece Taylor was among a large group who traveled to Abaco, The Bahamas, for a spring mission trip to help with the continuing clean-up and restoration needed after Hurricane Dorian destroyed the small community. Pictures of this largely college-aged group trickled back via social media. Seeing them working, laughing, playing with the children, and worshiping as a team filled my heart. Taylor would later tell me it was one of the most incredible experiences of her life. A small group within a larger community helping others to heal.

My experience at church has been so much better because of the influence of these young people. They are energetic and ready to take on the world for their King.

The prayer I scribbled on that note card several months ago has been put in motion. I prayed for faith like theirs. Faith that would allow me to be brave. One after another, their actions of faith have inspired me to trust in the prayers of strangers and the goodness of my God. I hope I was able to help some of their prayers be answered as well.

Wading In: Who inspires you?

Deep Dive: Share your thanks by writing a note or providing a meal.

Crowding Out For Fellowship

As I've shared (over and over again) throughout this chapter, I love people and cooking. Dinner parties are probably my favorite gathering, and I've reached a level of practical experience where I feel comfortable inviting guests to join us with short- notice. Even though I consider hosting one of my gifts, I've had moments where I dismiss the idea and close off my house to friends because I'm tired or the bathrooms need cleaning. Or maybe I don't have the energy or ingredients to serve a worthy meal. Jeff will often coerce me to extend the invitation, promising to help (how does mowing the grass help me in the kitchen?), and I give in.

In the past, I thought creating space for community meant I had to host in my freshly cleaned house with home-cooked food. The everything-cooked-from-scratch-on-the-day phase lasted long enough for me to tire of missing out on social time while I finished cooking or doing dishes. I found myself resenting the fun others had when we gathered, and I picked fights in the middle of the meal with "he who mows the lawn."

I neglected to consider that a gathering didn't have to be premeditated or extravagant. Community doesn't have a set menu, an ideal number of participants, or even a specific purpose.

The following list may have been born out of frustration, but relaxing my previous standards has served me well!

1 Minute:

- Extend an invitation: Make the call. Send a group text. Start the ball rolling and see if someone else will join you
- Respond to an invitation: Follow up with someone who has invited you!

- Drop off: Take a plate of cookies or a container of soup to someone in your neighborhood.

5- 10 Minutes:

- Initiate the idea: Create a FaceBook group or group chat. Ask a small group to meet.
- Visit at the fence: Many people don't know their neighbors! Make the excuse of admiring their roses and introduce yourself!
- Take a lap: Take a walk around the block. Say hello to everyone you meet. Your new best friend might live half a block away!

30 Minutes:

- Meet for coffee: See the same cars in the pick-up line day after day? Hop out of your vehicle and suggest an afternoon coffee with other moms.
- Lunch in motion: Meet with coworkers for a walk at lunchtime. Bonus points if you have a focused conversation about a book you're reading (rather than grumbling about work)

60-90 minutes:

- Book Club: Read a great book? Take the lead and suggest it to your friends! Coordinate a meeting date and provide snacks. Ask one of your friends to pick the next book and let them take responsibility for planning that event. It might have been your idea in the first place, but release some of the responsibility to others. They become more vested in the group when they're helping out.
- Lunch: Sometimes, groups are so action-oriented that they forget to gather to reflect on the good things they do (or the things that can improve). Step away from doing and enjoy conversation with the people you work with.
- Class time: Invite your friends to a class where none of you are the "expert." Enjoy the opportunity to learn together. It could be a class on prayer, crafts, or wine tasting- anything will do. New learners like to share, naturally forming a bond between participants.

- Playdate: Can't find a babysitter? Go out on a limb and ask some moms or caregivers you know to meet at a park or the pool.

2 Hours:

- Dinner Party: Make a plan. Make it simple. I like to cook one large, hands-off protein and offer a variety of salads and sides. I almost always serve buffet style. Don't be afraid to order carry-out. The point is to enjoy time with others, not to win an *Iron Chef*[4] competition.
- Family picnic: Invite your family to meet at a park and let everyone bring food. Time together without the fuss!
- Community Potluck: Remember the good old days when the church would host a Potluck? I can still taste the tater tot casserole and strawberry pretzel salad! Take the initiative to gather some friends to organize an event!
- Freeze Party: Check out sites like The Family Freezer[5] for recipes that can be easily multiplied. Gather some girlfriends and divide the work! I did this a few times with my gym family. It's so much more fun to dice onions or chop chicken when you're with your friends! Split the costs, and everyone leaves with freezer meals to save you on a crazy day!

All Day:

- Reunion or Holiday:

  Create a plan! Determine when and where you would like to meet. Consider a day that's not an official holiday, and if you want to guarantee a large group, begin planning months in advance.

  Ask for help. Offer to cook a portion of the meal and assign others to bring specific food items or to provide plates and cups. Don't forget about ordering takeout and giving everyone the chance to contribute.

  Extend grace. There is a good chance some people will say they will attend and won't show up. Or maybe they won't respond to the invitation. Rather than getting mad, check in on them, let them know they were missed, and extend an invitation for next time.

I can't believe I'm admitting this in a public forum, but through crowding out and creating time for people, I realized that mowing the lawn was just an excuse to stay out of my way while I was trying to "do it all." I'm thankful for Jeff's nudge to bring people to the table. We've reached a happy place where I cook, and he cleans up after, and we both get to enjoy a gathering of friends at home.

That being said, there are only twenty-four hours in a day.

If your life is like mine, you've likely tried to borrow a few more hours for today from tomorrow on more than one occasion. It's never worked for me, so if you figure it out, give me a shout!

I've learned that everything on my to-do list will be there tomorrow, but there is a chance that the people I love won't be.

The current trend is to protect your time. To say no. To shun the guilt of declining another invitation. I hope the trend will pass as soon as possible.

We're created to be in community. It doesn't matter what the house looks like or what's on the menu; send the invitation. Spend time with people. Organize a BBQ or a potluck- you don't have to do it alone. Ask some friends to join you for a walk. Join a book group. Volunteer at a local event.

Share your stories. Share your love. Do it often, and the world will be a better place.

"For where two or three come together in my name, I am there with them."

Matthew 18:20 NIRV

♥

Chapter 7

Let Go

For Fun

Walking on the beach, I noticed an abundance of broken shells… the outer portions of many were chipped away and polished to resemble a flower. Broken but beautiful. It would appear the usefulness of the shell was complete as it was no longer a safe harbor, but in this new form, it still brought me great joy.

It occurred to me that our lives are similar. We may have worked as moms or nurses, teachers or cashiers, high-powered CEOs, or small business owners. At the end of our careers, without the weight of our former identity, we're allowed to shed our shells and become something new.

We don't give a second thought to providing our children an opportunity to try new things. I don't remember discussing the return on investment when my sons wanted to try a new sport, sing in the choir, or take an art class. I happily purchased clarinets, soccer shoes, golf clubs, and cameras so they could experience new things and explore their passions.

My creative energy during those early years of motherhood was spent packing lunches and coordinating schedules so everyone could be where they were supposed to be when they were supposed to be there.

I watched my oldest son participate in activities for many years. I was running a restaurant back then, and my scheduled hours kept me on my feet, so watching Zachary was a chance to stop and rest. I was able to reduce my hours to part-time later in life, so I tagged along when my youngest started Tae Kwon Do, choosing movement instead of watching. I enjoyed it, but once Sam stopped attending, I did too.

The next time I did something for myself, it was in the wee hours of the morning, so I could accommodate everyone else's schedule! I worked out for several years before the sun rose so I could manage things for my guys at home.

Since the boys have grown and moved away, I've taken various creative classes, including photography, knitting, and clay throwing. I've participated in beginner Tai Chi and yoga. I've splurged to attend workshops and conferences to develop the confidence to pursue my love of writing. I've also invested in year-long certifications to be a better nutritionist and health coach.

I have to be honest. I've often doubted myself. I'm not an educated woman in the traditional sense; the pressures of working a full-time job outweighed my ability to get out of bed for class during my brief stint in college.

On surveys, I would check the box that said "some college" rather than marking "high school diploma" to make myself feel better. I've often wondered why there isn't a "life experience" option.

I've worked hard to make up for the lack of a degree; I became a proficient researcher, reading anything I could get my hands on to solve a problem. My sons often joke that I know things no one else even considers! I listen intently in church, I am a believer in lifelong learning, and I've learned to trust my gut.

Thirteen years ago, while managing my husband's business office, I started working part-time at the gym I attended. My job as a coach was to cheer on the members who worked out when I did and to chase them down if they missed a class or two. I was their accountability partner, and I loved it.

As a former restaurant manager and mother of active boys, this responsibility was in my wheelhouse; encouraging others as they moved toward health was a natural fit, and I worked to be the best coach I could be. My gut told me I had something more to offer as a coach and instructor. Somehow, by God's grace and my family's support, we made it happen. I sought out a business I respected, trained with my franchisors, studied to complete certifications, and worked to help others learn how to change their lives and enjoy fitness.

When I closed the doors to the gym, I thought my career was over because I would no longer see clients. But there was a longing forming in the absence of a job. I started to notice more and more opportunities to share my story and the stories of the men and women who inspired me. This book was slowly evolving in my mind.

As I considered writing, my doubting brain said I had no right, but my gut whispered that thousands of women in this world need to hear what I have to say.

Writing has been a dream of mine for a long time; I have journals full of ideas and outlines and great titles! But until I took the first step, allowing myself to attend an online conference, I never imagined I could write 60,000 purposeful words in my lifetime, little less 60,000 words between the covers of one book.

If you're reading this and you feel like your life is lacking purpose or if your mission is complete, I'd like to challenge you to find a new passion. So much of what we dream remains unwritten, unpainted… incomplete. Treat your passions as gifts for those you love and get them into the world!

Set your intention every day to do two things: share your joy with someone and find happiness for yourself. If you do this day after day, you will find a new purpose and, who knows, maybe a new career or adventure.

Trust your gut. And find your way.

Let Go of Insecurities

Wading In: List things you love to do "for fun."

Deep Dive: How can you share these passions with the world?

♥

Gifts

"Each of you should use whatever gift you have received to serve others, as faithful stewards of God's grace in its various forms."

1 Peter 4:10

My gifts are cooking and cheering people on. I used those talents in my younger years managing a restaurant. I prided myself on stepping into any position to complete the chain required each day to serve our customers. I tried to make work fun for my staff and was lucky to retain great employees during my years at that job.

I used those same gifts in my home when the boys were growing up. Cooking and cheering them on- trying to create an environment in our home that they wanted to share with their friends and would like to return to as they grew older. Once the boys became self-sufficient and my short-order cook services were no longer needed as often, it felt right to make a career change. The gym and coaching evolved naturally out of the things I did best.

My gym was manned solely by a dedicated team of volunteers. We operated on a foundation of shared passion and purpose, introducing countless individuals to the excitement of group fitness and challenge-based programs. Instructors, coaches, and cheerleaders - each person contributed their unique gifts to our vibrant community, and over time, they became like an extension of my own family. Some discovered a love for fitness through this journey and worked to obtain their own certifications.

Kaylen was one of those team members who could be counted on to rise to the occasion every time it was offered. She loved working out, being fit, and the community at my gym.

It was her smile I was drawn to first; big and bright, pushing her cheeks into her eyes so she squinted- she was constantly squinting because she was always smiling. Kaylen was upbeat and more full of joy than anyone I've ever known.

I met her the day before her challenge started. We'd emailed back and forth a few times about the gym facilities because she lived out of town and needed to be able to get ready for work after class. We scheduled an appointment, and I remember feeling sad I would have to turn her away because the shower remodel would not be ready before her session started.

She walked in, and before I could sugarcoat my news, she informed me, quite matter-of-factly, that she'd found a solution and would see me the following day at testing. This was the first of many experiences where I witnessed her can-do attitude rise above all obstacles to make things right.

She was a determined challenger and eventually became one of my team members, first as a coach and then as an instructor. She embraced everything we offered, including cross-training, yoga, and, eventually, weightlifting with our trainer.

She was Canadian by birth and Iowan via marriage. I often thought about how hard it would be to uproot life, moving away from everything (and everyone) I had ever known. She became a treasured friend, and I often admired all she did to help others.

She supported her new family in their hobbies at state and county fairs, raised money for Cystic Fibrosis to support her stepson, and drove long hours back and forth to Manitoba each year to stay entrenched in the lives of her family.

As the years passed, her passion for weightlifting increased, and she found her way to a new gym a few times a week. She would meet with a trainer who would give her workouts to complete in between sessions. She was determined to be stronger than ever- this new hobby became a passion, and she wanted all she could get.

Kaylen was always sparked by a challenge, and she pushed herself to swallow her doubts and train for a powerlifting competition. I remember creating "Team Kaylen" shirts with a few other friends as we prepared to support her in her first event.

Focus. Breathe. LIFT. Smile; this was her rhythm.

She was terrific, and it was evident she had found her place.

Sometime after I closed my gym, she moved a short distance away. I had the good fortune to meet her for lunch and was again amazed by her can-do attitude. She's still competing, recently at a national event, and she's started coaching young women in their quest to learn more about the sport (and themselves along the way) through the *Raise the Bar*[1] Initiative and their local high school Barbell Clubs.

She also works full-time, gathers with people to participate in curling and outdoor fun, and enjoys time with her faithful four-legged sidekick. I'm unsure where she finds the time to do it all, but I want to be like her when I grow up! Kaylen is a true testament to living life fully and using her passions to serve others. She is hungry for life and appears determined to experience as much of it as possible!

Let Go of Limitations- You Can Do Anything!

Wading In: What new thing would you like to try?

Deep Dive: What are your Gifts?
How can they open new doors for you?

♥

Head Nowhere

"Sometimes you find yourself in the middle of nowhere and sometimes in the middle of nowhere, you find yourself."

Stacy Westfall[2]

I set the cruise control, and I said a prayer, "Please don't let me regret this, Lord. I know there's a shorter way, but I might never have this opportunity again. Guide me. Protect me. See me safely home."

I'd said these exact words numerous times over the last few days, and at one point in my preparation, I was confident He would see me through. Now that the journey had begun, I wondered if I was up to the challenge ahead.

Jeff and I spent the previous month in Scottsdale, Arizona. It was our trial run at snow-birding, although in September, it's still beautiful in Iowa and hot in Arizona! During that month, we realized we could indeed move life to a temporary destination for a month or two. He worked, I wrapped up an online course, and we had a great time. We enjoyed the sun and sites with family members who visited, but Jeff was called out of town for business near the end of our stay. His itinerary should have had him back in time for us to drive home together, but at the last minute, his return was delayed.

I was confident in my ability to drive, but I'd never gone that far by myself! Most of our vacations in the past were within four hours from home or reached by plane because of our schedules.

When the pandemic grounded the world, we discovered how much we enjoyed a good old road trip. Jeff and I travel well together; he drives, and I chart the course. We listen to talk radio and sing along to the oldies when we get tired. We eat lunch out of a cooler and plan where we want to stop for the night. More often than not, we're done for the day before the sun goes down.

Several years ago, my husband suffered complications from a spinal surgery that caused his right diaphragm to become paralyzed. He has some difficulty breathing, and we avoid high altitudes when we're traveling. We'd driven in the southwest several times but usually followed a southern route, trekking through New Mexico and Texas before moving north toward home.

We briefly discussed the idea of me checking into a hotel to wait for him to fly back, but after looking at a map, I decided to swallow my doubt and take the long way home.

Because I was driving solo on this trip, I plotted my course north out of Arizona. I'd heard about the beautiful national parks scattered through Utah but had never seen them except out the window from 30,000 feet. On my first day, I chose a route that would take me through Monument Valley to Moab, Utah.

I was driving along, minding my own business, singing along with my favorite playlist, and suddenly, I rounded a bend and was in the middle of a valley I had only imagined! The rocks rose from the plains, artistically set like they had been staged on my behalf. Around every corner, there was something that took my breath away. I cried, and I prayed. I spent time standing in the middle of the road (with half a dozen other folks), camera in hand, because I knew I couldn't possibly remember the glory of it all. It was an incredible day.

From my journal that night:

"I left early, so I would be in Moab before dark like I promised! I traveled steadily north– my breath being taken from me again and again. I know these rocks and canyons have stood forever and ever, but somehow, it felt like they were created just for me. Swiping through my tears, I almost missed a sign pointing to a canyon overlook (which one? I don't know!) just south of here. I knew I was pushing against time, but I had to see... halfway down a twenty-mile trail. It dawned on me that I hadn't seen a car since the turn.

Anxiety began to creep in... was this a mistake?

Finally, I came upon a parking lot and other people. I climbed a few stairs up to the top of the rock, and suddenly, the world opened up into canyons of red and shadows of deep purple as far as my eye could see. A storm was in the distance, and the sun was streaming through the clouds. Magical... It was simply magical.

He was with me today. That's for sure. I felt the nudge to turn– it was so beautiful. I've never felt so small or been so caught up in His love. I'm exhausted, but can't wait to wake up tomorrow to catch the sunrise at Arches."

The next day, I woke in time to witness sunrise at Arches National Park and caught the sunset on the western edge of Nebraska.

In between those two points, I crossed the mountaintops of Colorado. With a death grip on the steering wheel and my foot on the brake, I managed to call Jeff twice and each boy once. I used the calls to distract myself from the task and tell them I loved them, just in case I flew over the edge while trying to keep up with traffic! I don't know how a person gets used to 70 mph downhill with nothing but a guardrail between them and eternity, but I'm sure I will never do it again! I also called on God no less than a hundred times, a few times to beg for protection but more often to offer praise for the creation all around me.

I arrived home on time, two and a half days after I left Scottsdale. I'm proud of how I set a plan and stuck to it (even if there was one pretty spectacular detour). I experienced incredible moments in the valley and conquered fear on the mountaintop. I proved to myself that I can achieve good things with a lot of prayer and patience. I can't wait to see where He leads me next.

Let Go of Fear.

Wading In: Where do you want to go?

Deep Dive: What do you hope to find there?

♥

Take the Time

"It's not how much we give,
but how much love we put into giving."

Mother Teresa[3]

Most of us believe it's our responsibility to give back once we've acquired a certain level of success or financial stability. Still, we often forget the impact we can make with our service in place of monetary contributions.

People can get caught up in a false valuation of their worth in a world that often emphasizes personal achievements and material gain. It's easy to convince yourself you're too busy to make a difference, write a check, and forget about it. But as much as I realize the importance of financial contributions, I think gifts of service are desperately needed and overlooked by most people as a way of giving back.

One of the true joys of life can be found in giving selflessly. When we share our time and talents with others, we tap into a wellspring of fulfillment and meaning that simply can't be measured by material possessions alone, and it reflects in the kind of people we become.

She always calls me Kimmie. No one has ever called me Kimmie except my grandparents, God bless their souls, and Susan. Somehow, when she says it, it feels right, like she's excited to see me, and I like that. She's the kindest person I know, loving, giving, in touch with the needs of others, and ultimately "go with the flow."

Susan is also an old soul. By definition, that means someone who demonstrates a maturity or understanding of one much older. She writes snail mail cards, visits people even if it's inconvenient for her, and loves her family with an inspiring fierceness. She forgives without thought and remembers others even when she's been forgotten. I've witnessed her "offer the other cheek" time and time again.

She has one of those jobs I'm envious of. She works hard, often helping people at their lowest when they've experienced a loss or been in an accident, and her company allows her time to volunteer. Most people grumble about the requirement to spend a Friday afternoon helping at a food bank or serving various organizations in the community, but not Susan. She shares stories of the people she meets and has become a friend to many. She's a living example of how giving our time allows us to form genuine connections with others.

Dan Buettner, author of *The Blue Zone*, states, "Altruism stimulates the same neural pathways as sugar and cocaine. But unlike drugs, volunteering is a healthy addiction. People who volunteer tend to lose weight, have lower rates of heart disease, and report higher levels of happiness. Decide what you do best and volunteer your time."[4]

Volunteering at community centers, shelters, or retirement homes provides an opportunity to engage with individuals from diverse backgrounds, fostering empathy and understanding. These connections not only enrich our lives but also enhance the social fabric of our communities.

Selflessly giving our time opens doors to personal growth and self-discovery. It allows us to step outside our comfort zones, acquire new skills, and gain a deeper understanding of the world. In serving others, we often find that we achieve more than we give, as the act of giving expands our horizons and broadens our perspectives.

When we give our time and talents, we inspire those around us to do the same. Our acts of kindness and generosity can have a ripple effect, igniting a chain reaction of giving that spreads throughout our communities. Leading by example, we motivate others to make a difference.

Research has consistently shown that acts of giving improve personal well-being. Engaging in charitable activities has been linked to reduced stress levels, increased happiness, and improved mental health.

Through volunteer services of your choice, you can help your community and experience better health and well-being. There are countless opportunities to give back to meet the needs of our communities.

Let Go of Excuses. Your Time is Valuable!

Wading In: Who can you support today?

Deep Dive: Where is the gap in your community? How can you spark a movement?

Make the Change

Hey! Guess what? The sun that rises majestically over the ocean in Florida also rises in Iowa! Today, it rose precisely two hours and three minutes after I woke up and got tired of watching the fan spin above my head. I'm unsure if it's hormones or a deadline that's nudged me up today, but here I am, watching the sky turn pink out my office window.

I found health and God and joy again last winter, all by myself in the wee hours of the morning. I would sneak out of bed to write and pray. I prioritized my schedule so I could lace my tennies and be out the door just as the color started to fill the sky.

Instead of letting the aches and pains of "old age" tell me what I could do, I chose what my body would do. In the process of taking charge, my body changed.

Back at home (also known as the real world), I allowed some old habits to get in the way. Cold mornings beckoned me to hit the snooze bar, and I quit prioritizing time for myself. Somehow, the days fly by quicker when I have a to-do list and agenda filled with other people's plans.

But that's my fault, isn't it? During the months when I was away from home, I placed my needs equal to those of others, and my commitments were easily rearranged to allow exercise and healthy cooking. I didn't allow the comfort of a warm bed to disrupt my plan or my time outside. And I didn't let a busy day push my health aside.

Have you ever thought about how blessed you are?

I think about it a lot. Three months of "snowbirding" in a warmer climate proved I'm not too old to get in shape.

Sure, I have aches and pains and days when I audibly creak climbing out of a chair. But isn't it better to be sore because I'm working to improve my health rather than sitting too long in that chair? My flexibility is returning, but not without discomfort. I'm sleeping better, but not without an intentional routine. My internal markers are improving because I'm focusing on real food. I'm returning to a healthier version of me, one decision at a time.

Like so many women in middle age, I had resigned to the fact that I couldn't achieve the health of my younger years. I believed it when someone said my hormones would determine my weight. Menopause belly, brain fog, and fatigue are all just excuses. Has my body changed? Yes. Do I have to accept it? No.

I'm tired of the people in my world putting limitations on what I can do because of my age. I'm sure I'll never run a marathon in my lifetime, not because I can't but because I don't want to. Maybe I'll lift heavy things or learn to row or snowshoe- all I know is that whatever I choose to do, I will do it because it brings me joy.

This decision to be healthy has the opportunity to cause some angst in the lives around me. I won't settle for "you're too old" or "it's your age." If I'm willing to put forth the effort, those around me can either join in or sit back and watch. I can't worry about what the world thinks anymore because I'm running out of time, and I have a lot of things remaining on my bucket list!!

This process requires me to be my own advocate. I've been able to watch people I love very much be offered the band-aids of medication when what they really needed was the readjustment of sharp words. Some diseases are age-related, and some are genetic, *but of the top five killers* (cancer, cardiovascular disease, COPD, diabetes, and stroke), 80% are caused by lifestyle factors.[5]

Look for doctors who are honest with you. Prevention is the key to a long life, and most of us didn't do an excellent job preventing it when we were younger. If you don't feel good physically, mentally, emotionally, or spiritually, find help. But please don't accept a pill as your only answer. Medications are great for short-term assistance, but most drugs were not created for lifelong consumption. Ask your provider how you can work to reduce your need for medication; create a plan with their help and test for progress as often as your insurance will allow.

A report published by the Center for Disease Control[6] in 2019 states that nearly seven in ten adults in the US and Canada aged forty to seventy-nine used at least one prescription drug in the past thirty days, and around one in five used at least five prescription drugs.

Among adults aged forty to fifty-nine, the most commonly used prescriptions were antidepressants, drugs for lowering cholesterol or blood pressure, and analgesics.

Curiously, the following lifestyle choices combine to alleviate the symptoms of the diseases managed by the prescriptions above:

Diet: Whole, unrefined, minimally processed, mostly plants helps reduce diabetes, heart disease, and cancer risk. Evidence shows that the Mediterranean diet can reduce the risk of developing cardiovascular disease and other chronic diseases. This diet is rich in vegetables, fruits, legumes, whole grains, fish, olive oil, and nuts.

Physical activity: Moving helps all your body's systems. Experts recommend 150 minutes of moderate-intensity activity each week. Simply move more and sit less.

Sleep: Try to get seven to nine hours of restful sleep each night. Have a consistent bedtime and wake time, even on the weekends. Limit alcohol and caffeine. Put digital devices away 90 minutes before bedtime. Keep your sleep area cool, dark, and comfortable.

Stress relief: Chronic stress is a major disruption to your immune system. Several practices mentioned in Chapter One can help bring your stress levels to a manageable place.

Social connectedness: Simply loving people can keep you emotionally and physically healthy.

We can blame any number of things as the cause of our conditions, but we live in a time of great abundance. Avoid the drive-thru in favor of a grocery store or fresh-air market. Disconnect from media in favor of activities with people you care about. Learn to be patient with yourself- changes happen quickly but are often difficult to spot. Keep going! Get used to feeling good!

Let Go of the Status Quo.

Wading In: List your medications. Which one could be "worked" away?

Deep Dive: How can you take active steps to change your health?

Relax

It's 5:00 somewhere, right?

When I was a girl, I always told myself I would never smoke and would never drink. Both habits were stinky and "bad." I didn't *know* this to be true because they weren't teaching about it yet in school, and I couldn't google it, but my personal experiences told me so. I grew up during a time when cigarette smoking was widely accepted. Grocery stores and doctors' offices had ashtrays in them, airplanes and restaurants had smoking sections, and because my dad smoked, we often sat in those sections. Drinking was bad because it made my parents fight.

I smoked my first cigarette when I was fifteen. We had just moved to a new town, I was acting like a brat (see chapter one), and a lot of the kids at school were smoking other substances. Cigarettes seemed safer than pot, so I did that for a while. I battled back and forth with smoking for several years, quitting just shy of my fortieth birthday. I hit the pause button with each pregnancy, but the lure of "stress relief" pulled me back time and time again. Giving up smoking was by far the hardest thing I've ever done until now.

I didn't drink alcohol regularly until my late twenties. I'd had a few drinks here and there, but I was afraid I would have a problem based on my family history. Several members of my family have struggled with addiction, and I didn't want to follow down the same road.

I've had fewer beers than I can count on my right hand, and hard liquor seems to guarantee I'm going to sleep in a spinning room. As it turns out, I like wine. My consumption has ranged from an occasional glass to a bottle a night, depending on the state of many things. Unfortunately, drinking is a pastime widely accepted in my circle of friends, and the reason to drink could vary from celebrating to commiserating (to everything in between).

I quit drinking a few times to achieve weight loss goals, but after explaining myself time and time again, it didn't seem worth it. Tell someone you're not drinking, and they look at you like you're sick, you're crazy, or you have a *real* problem.

The first time I considered I might be drinking out of habit rather than choice, I joined the online group *Sober Sis*[7]. I met several women trying to cut back, and a few of us became fast friends as we shared our struggles. It was nice to work through why I wanted a drink every night at 5:00 pm with someone who wasn't sitting across a table. It felt anonymous and safe.

After a great deal of self-examination, I learned I had trained myself to need a glass of wine. My work day didn't end, and my stressors didn't go away until the smooth, sweet liquid crossed my lips. My wine of choice is a California cabernet, readily available nationwide for the reasonable price of fifteen dollars a bottle. I often tried other wines, regions, and varieties, only to be disappointed with the taste. If I wasn't at home and couldn't have a glass of my favorite (or something very similar), I would drink water instead of another kind of drink.

I reassured myself that my habit seemed to be influenced more by a "taste" than a physical need (but that still doesn't mean it is good for me). Many women I met during the Sober Sis 21-day challenge sought substitutes for their drink of choice; the beer drinkers were often satisfied with non-alcoholic beers, and the liquor drinkers could usually find a substitute, even if it wasn't quite right. Fortunately for me, the red wine alternatives are generally terrible. I'm confident I wouldn't have been able to break my "taste addiction" if I had found an acceptable replacement.

I started experimenting with mocktails to occupy my time and satisfy my taste buds. It fits into my skill set to experiment with food, so why not drinks as well? I've included several recipes in the Back of the Book. Let me know if you try one or create your own! I'm always up for a new recipe!

Many assume the occasional beer or glass of wine at mealtimes or special occasions doesn't pose much cause for concern. But, drinking any amount of alcohol can potentially lead to unwanted health consequences. People who binge drink or drink heavily may notice more health effects sooner, but alcohol also poses some risks for people who drink in moderation.

Many of us know the temporary effects of drinking, which include positive feelings of relaxation or drowsiness, mood changes, and lowered inhibitions, but also unwanted effects of slurred speech, vomiting, or loss of decision-making or consciousness.

Long-term effects of alcohol use can cause persistent changes in mood, including anxiety, insomnia, a weakened immune system, problems with memory, and increased tension in relationships.

If you think you might need to take a step back from drinking or many other substances, you have plenty of options for support and treatment:

- free recovery support groups, like *Alcoholics Anonymous*[8] or *Celebrate Recovery*[9]
- online recovery platforms and coaching, like Sober Sis or *Ditched the Drink*[10]
- therapy to help address reasons for drinking and learn helpful coping skills
- medical treatment
- The *Substance Abuse and Mental Health Services Administration* offers a free helpline, available 24/7. Call 800-662-HELP (4357) or TTY 1-800-487-4889 to get guidance on local options for support and treatment.[11]

I recently went more than three months without wine, and I didn't miss it. I lost weight and felt great. I reduced bloat around my middle, and my psoriasis cleared. I slept better, wrote better, exercised more regularly, and thankfully had no withdrawal symptoms. I've raised my lemon water or cranberry shrub and soda at more than a few celebration meals and it seems to be okay!

Let Go of Numbing.

Wading In: Make a list of healthy ways to relax.

Deep Dive: What about your day do you need to escape?

Just Right

Writing a book has been a process like no other I've ever experienced. If you were my friend, I'd gladly sit down with you and share my stories and experiences, but somehow, the permanence of writing things down has me spiraling into a quest for words.

I haven't used a thesaurus since I was in high school. I checked and rechecked my facts to ensure I was sharing the truth with you. I had long conversations with friends and sent my chapters to experts in my desire to "do no harm."

Over the last few weeks, everyone I've talked to has asked me, "How's it Going?" Those three words have become the bane of my existence, and until this morning, I couldn't figure out why.

My words weren't flowing because I was searching for perfection. Up to this point, I've repeatedly told you there is no perfect in this world- no perfect diet, exercise plan, or prayer routine. Yet, I have been avoiding my computer because I couldn't find the perfect words to wrap this up.

I struggled to finish because I wanted it to be "just right." To be perfect, but if it was perfect, it would only work for me.

I realize this small book will likely never reach masterpiece status, so why not just put my experiences and stories on the page and pray that my heart's words will help you somehow? Maybe you'll laugh. Maybe you'll cry. Maybe you'll eat a few more vegetables or cook a few more meals at home. Maybe my book will land in the hands of a woman who is ready to give up, and through my ramblings, she finds hope.

There are no perfect words, foods, or plans, but there are many perfect components to put together a life full of health and joy.

Pictures of my perfect things hang on my walls and line my bookcases. They fill my journals and sweetly haunt my memories. They taste like childhood treats, filling my heart with so much emotion I can't help but cry.

I intended to share stories and actions that have worked for me to give you hope as you chart your journey toward health.

To be healthy, you need to do some basic things:

- You need to eat wholesome food. Wholesome food comes from plants or pastures, ocean or stream. It has minimal ingredients and shouldn't need a label.
- You need to move your body. Raise your heart rate, challenge your strength, and stretch your muscles. Every day, in some way.
- You need to drink water.
- You need to rest. Mind, body, and soul.
- You need to gather with other people. Share stories, make new memories, and have fun.
- You need to believe in something greater than yourself.
- You need to have a purpose- challenge yourself to be a little better every day.
- Learn. Love. Explore. Volunteer.

Live your life from a place of wonder and gratitude and experience great joy.

Let Go of Perfection.

Wading In: Who's imperfect life inspires you?

Deep Dive: Who needs your joyful example of imperfection?

♥

Crowding Out for Yourself

So many of the tools I would offer you in this chapter are already scattered throughout the book:

Breathe. Pray. Write. Dream. Move your body.
Eat good food. Spend time with friends.

The problem is that you already know this, but you'll never live the life you were meant to live until you let go of society's demands and your own expectations. So, in this chapter, I offer one tool:

Turn it Around

Learn to identify the negative talk and the doubts in your life. You can do it because you likely notice it when someone drones on about how awful their life is. Every cloud has a silver lining, right? Find it. Write it down. Again and again and again.

Do it until you no longer see the bad in the world but opportunities to help.

Do it until you no longer dread the job but enjoy the connection with your co-workers.

Do it until you no longer look in the mirror and feel ashamed but acknowledge the progress.

Do it until others notice a change in you and begin to look at the world in a new way.

Let go of what was and be the spark that makes the world better.

Conclusion

You Decide

It Can Be Easy

Being healthy is easy- I hope I showed you it can also be enjoyable. It may not be the norm- your families will protest for a while. Your friends will look in your cart at the grocery store and think, "What is she going to do with all those vegetables?" People are going to throw things at you like "You're such a good cook," or "You're so devoted to your routine," or better yet, "You take such good care of us."

Being healthy is easy- it's how most of us entered this world: healthy, screaming, and kicking our feet. We hollered when we were hungry and stretched when we woke. We toddled into years when we became self-sufficient at things like eating and moving. How amazing to shove smooshed carrots into our mouths and scoot along the floor, working to that incredible moment when our legs held us up, and we learned to run. We were born with the desire to move.

Being healthy is easy- we're created to be happy, free of stress, and content to be hopelessly dependent on someone to comfort us. We slept when we were tired and learned the joy of snuggling up with the ones who loved us.

Being healthy is easy- it's our self-regulating birthright. It's our God-given instinct to do the things that make us whole. Eat when you're hungry, move when you're awake, explore the world around you, love the ones who care for you, trust the ones who created you, and believe in the wonder of the One who created it all.

Being healthy is easy… but pushing back against well-meaning parents who just need you on a schedule, schools following classroom guidelines, or friends who "just want to chill" is hard. And breaking a lifetime of habits is hard.

I watched over a thousand people change their lives with my former method. Thousands of people lost tens of thousands of pounds by changing their diets and moving their bodies. But if I polled them today, I'd guess many have gained it all back, plus more.

We've been conditioned to think that a healthy life has to be complicated; healthy food will taste bad, and healthy movement will hurt our aging bodies.

I hope I've shown you none of those beliefs are true.

You Can Make it Hard

I recently completed a challenge ominously named *"75Hard"*.[1] My publisher threw the idea out during our cohort's weekly check-in. He was going to start at the beginning of the new year and offered us the accountability of a group.

I did some research because the name indicated it was everything I've been running from for the last several years (by now, you've figured out I'm anti-hard). The founder of this self-regulated list of tasks created the plan to reach a fitness goal. Throughout his experience, he discovered the psychological benefits of discipline were advantageous in many ways. His all-or-nothing approach still seemed restrictive: check the boxes daily. Miss a day = start over.

Workout twice a day for forty-five minutes, once outside

Drink a gallon of water

Take a progress picture

Read ten pages of a non-fiction book

Follow a diet

No cheat meals or alcohol

After talking it over and discussing how we would accomplish the tasks, Jeff and I decided this would be a great activity to share as we set out on our first official "snowbird" excursion. With three months of great weather guaranteed, why not do our best to better ourselves?

What I learned was my body responded quickly to good things: fresh air, good food, water, and movement. The fog hovering around my brain followed suit, lifting quickly with the reduction in sugar and alcohol and the addition of sleep. It was easier to process what I read, and the evidence of my efforts soon showed up in my photos.

Discipline differs from deprivation, and trusting someone else to establish the guidelines made me more prone to follow through. I enjoyed the experience and pushed toward the seventy-sixth day without agony.

Now that it's over, I'll continue in the following ways:

Workout twice daily for forty-five minutes, once outside: I was fortunate enough to be in a warm, sunny climate. I often walked both workouts, but if you remember, a workout can be endurance, strength, balance, or flexibility-based. If you don't belong to a gym, set up a space to move in your bedroom or the garage. Open the door to let the fresh air in and grab a jump rope, do a Tabata, or lift some weights. There are no space or equipment requirements- just move.

I'll continue to do one workout that fits the above criteria and take a walk sometime each day. I've discovered I do my best thinking and praying while my body is moving- it's the most wonderful form of multitasking!

Don't be afraid to leave the earbuds at home if you're walking alone. Enjoy the sound of the ocean or the ripple of the wind through the trees, the birds talking to one another, or the buzz of the bees. Breathe in deeply. Notice the smell of fresh air and walk. Remember to take a tape recorder or use a notes app on your phone to record the wonderful ideas that arise when you spend time in nature, in silence.

Drink a gallon of water: After completing the challenge, I backed off this one. A gallon is a lot, and I'm a fifty-five-year-old woman with pelvic-floor opportunities! I've settled in at eighty ounces on a typical day, more if it's terribly hot or my workout is particularly strenuous.

I listen to my body and drink regularly, trying to avoid moments of thirst.

Take a progress picture: not every day, but every week. It's nice to see changes in the mirror- a picture proves to yourself that you weren't imagining how great you look!

Read ten pages of a non-fiction book: I blow this away daily because I like learning. Ten pages often becomes a chapter or two. I read to learn early in the day and added reading for pleasure (always a traditional ink and paper book) to fill my soul and ease into sleep before bed.

Follow a diet: the diet I follow is mine- protein, carbs, fat, and veggies 90% of the time. I'll move forward with treats or alcohol no more than once or twice a week and eat home-cooked meals as often as possible.

No cheat meals or alcohol: see above. Long gone are the days when I'd pass on a piece of birthday cake or a glass of good wine when sharing a meal with friends. And goodbye to the guilt associated with cheat meals. I have treat meals, but only once in a while. I'll never again consume indulgent foods without the pleasure of time, taste, or quality. Life is too short to settle for mediocre food.

And never again will I say "everything in moderation." Moderation seems to be the slippery slope my bad habits are built on. The belief that "any food or drink once in a while" is a healthy position to take, but I also believe a little of *anything daily* has the opportunity to become a habit in the long run. I try to keep some variety in my indulgences because if I don't, I'll find myself mindlessly driving to the grocery at 8 pm because I'm out of crispy, crunchy snacks (the ones that leave your fingers orange), and my day can't be complete without just a few.

Being healthy is easy if you start healthy, but most of us aren't. So, choose a small action every day to get you back there. Count on others to help you and turn to God when others can't. Look for the good in everything. Count your blessings and say thank you when you're surprised. Look people in the eye. Smile. Eat, move, sleep, love, give, and learn.

There is no timeline, and the prize is guaranteed.

My Prayer for You

Dear God,

We come before you today with grateful hearts, acknowledging that being healthy is not always an easy journey. We confess that many of us have strayed from the path of good physical and spiritual health. But we know that with your guidance and the support of others, we can find our way back to a state of well-being.

Lord, help us choose small daily actions that will lead us towards a healthier life. Show us the steps we need to take, the habits we need to form, and the mindset we need to embrace. Give us the strength to make these choices consistently, even when it feels challenging.

Help us, O Lord, to see the good in everything surrounding us. Open our eyes to the blessings we often overlook and grant us the wisdom to express our gratitude. May we cultivate a spirit of thankfulness, acknowledging your grace and mercy. When surprises come our way, let us respond with heartfelt appreciation and praise.

Teach us to be present in our interactions with others, to truly see and connect with them. Grant us the ability to look people in the eye, offering them genuine love and kindness. Help us to be a source of encouragement and support for those around us, knowing that we are all on this journey together.

As we nourish our bodies, may we make wise choices in what we eat and drink. Guide us in finding the right balance between indulgence and self-discipline. Inspire us to move our bodies, exercise, and care for the temples you have given us. Grant us restful sleep, allowing our bodies and minds to rejuvenate.

Lord, teach us to love unconditionally, to extend grace and forgiveness to ourselves and others. May we be channels of your love, reaching out to those in need, offering a helping hand and a listening ear. Help us to learn and grow continually, expanding our knowledge and understanding of your world.

We know that on this journey towards health, there is no timeline. Yet we trust in your perfect timing and know that the prize of well-being is possible. Help us to remain steadfast, keeping our eyes fixed on you and the abundant life you promise.

Thank you for loving us,

Amen

The Back of the Book

This is where the good stuff lives!

KIM'S 55TH BLESSING LIST

From my journal: Saturday, December Tenth.

Happy Birthday to me! Fifty-five celebrations. Fifty-five years of learning, joy, hurt, doubt, and love. For every ebb, there has been a flow, and for them all, I am grateful. Through them, I have become the woman I am today. So, in a quest to make the day about more than cards and cake and Facebook messages, a fast list of things I'm thankful for in no particular order of importance because blessings are blessings ♥

1. Mom
2. Dad
3. Jeff
4. Zach
5. Sam
6. Kat
7. Madi
8. Grandparents
9. Dad
10. Christine
11. Teachers
12. Coaches
13. God The Father
14. Jesus-savior
15. Spirit-within
16. Books
17. A good steak
18. Old friends (Facebook!)
19. New friends
20. Smooth pens
21. Snail mail
22. Comfy shoes
23. Bear
24. Nash
25. Good pillows
26. Sisters
27. Brothers
28. Cousins

29. Aunts
30. Uncles
31. Reliable car
32. Candles
33. Sunrise
34. Oceans
35. Freshly mowed grass
36. New journals
37. Queso
38. Mountains
39. Ministers
40. Mentors
41. Google docs
42. Prayer
43. Fresh picked apple
44. Dark red wine
45. Christmas lights
46. Music
47. Road trips
48. My camera
49. Flowers
50. Clean towels
51. Fire
52. Chocolate
53. Autumn leaves
54. great haircuts
55. Snow

Thanks to God for a lifetime of good, sprinkled with enough sad and bad to make it real… for the love I've received and the good I've witnessed. Please grant me more years to share my blessings with others. *Amen*

EXAMPLE OF WRITTEN JOURNAL

Monday

5 am- Wake- 7 hours of sleep

Water w/ hydrant and 1 squirt Stur and 2 cups coffee (black)

9 am- Roasted sweet potato, mushrooms, sliced onion, handful spinach, 2 eggs, small handful blueberries, water

12 pm- Frozen cauliflower rice pilaf, ground beef, black beans, salsa, sharp cheddar, avocado, water

4 pm- ½ Kachava shake made with water

8 pm- Homemade black bean soup (with carrots, celery, peppers, turkey sausage), sour cream, raw celery, and carrots,

1 TOST beverage (delicious carbonated non-alcoholic cider-like beverage)

Walk 3 miles- total 88 oz. water

Tuesday

5:30 am- Wake- 7.5 hours of sleep

Water w/ hydrate and 1 squirt Stur and 2 cups coffee (black)

7 am- (hungry) Old-fashioned oats with half almond milk/half water, blueberries, 1 scoop protein powder, water

PROBIOTIC

11:30- (hungry) small apple w/ Peanut butter (had Jiff today- out of the natural fridge kind. It's been a long time... it was delicious!), water

2 pm- Bowl Black bean soup, pkt. Avocado mash, sour cream, Tostitos whole grain scoops □, water

6 pm- Chicken hindquarter (no skin), veggies (broccoli, zucchini, onion, mushrooms) sauteed in butter/chicken broth, water, and hot tea after dinner

8 pm- glass Cabernet

Walk 3 miles- 72 oz water

Wednesday

7:00- 9 hours sleep (didn't sleep well- wine is affecting me easier now)

Water w/ hydrate and 1 squirt Stur and 2 cups coffee (black)

10 am- 2 egg omelet with mushrooms and cheddar, small pear, hot water

PROBIOTIC

1:20 pm- small handful of diced chicken, cottage cheese, cherry tomatoes, celery, water

2:15- Treat- Tall caramel Macchiato w/ extra shot, water. Made me feel "off"- headache. Drank excess water to help it pass

6:30- Instant pot pasta (onion, pepper, mushrooms, 1 lb. local Italian sausage, 1 jar Muir Glen

pasta sauce, 1 box whole wheat rotini), fresh Mozzarella on top when served- delicious

Curious Elixir, water

Walk 3 miles- 80 oz. water

Thursday

7:10- 7 hours sleep. I read before bed and couldn't stop. Slept well, only woke once

Water w/ hydrate and 1 squirt Stur and 2 cups coffee (black)

2 pm- Chicken, whole grain bun, iced tea- I was starving! The meeting ran over, and this was the first chance to eat.

5 pm- Jeff and I met with friends. 3 oz wine (not familiar with any on the list- left half on the table- yuck), cheese, olives, pickle, summer sausage.

7 pm- Leftover pasta from last night- water

No exercise today- one of those days... 80 oz. water

Friday

6:00- 6 hours sleep. Early morning to get Jeff to the airport.

Water w/ hydrate and 1 squirt stur and 2 cups coffee (black)

7:15- Drive thru- venti Americano and protein box on the drive back home

11:45 am- Hungry! Last of the black bean soup with diced chicken, a sprinkle of cheddar, Tostitos, and grapes

5 pm- a handful of almonds, pecans, and chocolate chips- writing and wanting to finish the chapter.

9 pm- Hungry but don't feel like cooking a big meal. Scrambled eggs and toast

Sunrise on a different beach! Walk 2 miles- 100 oz. water

Saturday

4:30- 5 hours sleep. Woke early, want to have a good writing day

Water w/ hydrate and 1 squirt Stur and 2 cups coffee (black)

6:30- apple on walk

8:00- Plain Greek yogurt mixed with Noosa yogurt, berries, granola, coffee

2 pm- Turkey sandwich on thin bun, mayo, dijon, spinach, carrots, orange

7 pm- Egg roll in a bowl- glass + cabernet

9 pm- out! So tired!

Walk 3 miles- 80 oz. Water. Too much coffee... icky stomach this afternoon

Sunday

6:00- 8.5 hours sleep!

Water w/ hydrate and 1 squirt Stur and 2 cups coffee (black)

8:30- eggs, sourdough toast, jam

1 pm- Turkey sandwich on thin bun, mayo, dijon, spinach, celery/pb, pear.

6 pm- Mexican pot roast taco bowl, cauliflower rice, avocado, salsa, cheddar

8 pm- cinnamon tea,

Walk 4 miles-90 oz. water

EXAMPLE OF BULLET JOURNAL

Date: 4/24-30

Goals:

Water	☒ ☐ ☒ ☒ ☒ ☐ ☒
Write	☒ ☒ ☒ ☐ ☒ ☒ ☐
Walk	☒ ☒ ☒ ☒ ☒ ☒ ☐
Read	☒ ☐ ☒ ☒ ☒ ☐ ☒
	☐ ☐ ☐ ☐ ☐ ☐ ☐

Monday

Protein ☒ ☒ ☒ ☐ ☐ ☐

Fat ☒ ☒ ☐ ☐ ☐ ☐

Carbohydrates ☒ ☒ ☐ ☐ ☐ ☐

Vegetables ☒ ☒ ☒ ☒ ☒ ☐

Water ☒ ☒ ☒ ☒ ☒ ☒ ☒
☒ ☒ ☒ ☐ ☐ ☐ ☐

Other ☐ ☐ ☐ ☐ ☐ ☐ ☺

Tuesday

Protein ☒ ☒ ☒ ☒ ☐ ☐

Fat ☒ ☒ ☐ ☐ ☐ ☐

Carbohydrates ☒ ☐ ☐ ☐ ☐ ☐

Vegetables ☒ ☒ ☒ ☒ ☒ ☒

Water ☒ ☒ ☒ ☒ ☒ ☒ ☐
☐ ☐ ☐ ☐ ☐ ☐ ☐

Other ☒ ☐ ☐ ☐ ☐ ☐

Wednesday

Protein ☒ ☒ ☒ ☐ ☐ ☐

Fat ☒ ☒ ☒ ☐ ☐ ☐

Carbohydrates ☒ ☒ ☐ ☐ ☐ ☐

Vegetables ☒ ☒ ☒ ☒ ☒ ☐

Water ☒ ☒ ☒ ☒ ☒ ☒ ☒
☒ ☒ ☐ ☐ ☐ ☐ ☐

Other ☐ ☐ ☐ ☐ ☐ ☐

Thursday

Protein ☒ ☒ ☒ ☒ ☐ ☐

Fat ☒ ☒ ☒ ☒ ☐ ☐

Carbohydrates ☒ ☐ ☐ ☐ ☐ ☐

Vegetables ☒ ☒ ☒ ☒ ☐ ☐

Water ☒ ☒ ☒ ☒ ☒ ☒ ☒
☒ ☒ ☒ ☐ ☐ ☐ ☐

Other ☒ ☐ ☐ ☐ ☐ ☐

Friday

Protein ☒ ☒ ☒ ☒ ☐ ☐

Fat ☒ ☒ ☒ ☒ ☐ ☐

Carbohydrates ☒ ☒ ☐ ☐ ☐ ☐

Vegetables ☒ ☒ ☒ ☒ ☒ ☐

Water ☒ ☒ ☒ ☒ ☒ ☒ ☒
☒ ☐ ☐ ☐ ☐ ☐ ☐

Other ☒ ☐ ☐ ☐ ☐ ☐

Saturday

Protein ☒ ☒ ☐ ☐ ☐ ☐

Fat ☒ ☒ ☐ ☐ ☐ ☐

Carbohydrates ☒ ☒ ☐ ☐ ☐ ☐

Vegetables ☒ ☒ ☒ ☐ ☐ ☐

Water ☒ ☒ ☒ ☒ ☒ ☐ ☐
☐ ☐ ☐ ☐ ☐ ☐ ☐

Other ☒ ☐ ☐ ☐ ☐ ☐

Sunday

Protein ☒ ☒ ☒ ☒ ☐ ☐

Fat ☒ ☒ ☐ ☐ ☐ ☐

Carbohydrates ☒ ☒ ☒ ☐ ☐ ☐

Vegetables ☒ ☒ ☒ ☒ ☒ ☐

Water ☒ ☒ ☒ ☒ ☒ ☒ ☒
☒ ☐ ☐ ☐ ☐ ☐ ☐

Other ☒ ☒ ☐ ☐ ☐ ☐

MY FAVORITE FOODS

Proteins are the main building blocks in our bodies. There are several options but search for items that are minimally processed.

Poultry

Chicken: ground, bone-in, boneless, whole Eggs/ all-natural egg whites, Turkey: ground, bone-in, boneless, whole Wildfowl (duck, pheasant, grouse, quail)

Pork- ground, roast, loin, chops, Canadian bacon

Beef- ground, roast, steak

Wild Meats- bison, deer, elk: ground, roast, steak

Fish- Low-fat: cod, flounder, haddock, halibut, mahi mahi, orange roughy, tuna,

High-fat: anchovies, herring, mackerel, salmon, sardines. Look for wild-caught fish and check out seafoodwatch.com for clean, healthy choices.

If you live in the middle of the country with limited fresh fish options, check out a subscription service like wildalaskancompany.com. I've had great luck with this service!

Vegetarian Sources- You can find fresh edamame in the produce section, often still in the pod, but you can also find it already shelled. You can also buy frozen edamame with no additives.

Deli Meat- Keep to a minimum because of high sodium and hidden fats. Always choose "whole muscle" meats purchased at a deli counter over pre-packaged, processed meats in the refrigerated case if you need them.

Dairy- Cheese, cottage cheese, Greek yogurt

Protein Powders/Bars- Look for natural ingredients. Less is more here!

Carbohydrates

***Simple Carbohydrates* - fruits and veggies.** There are too many options to list! Fruits and veggies are high in antioxidants and fiber. They are a great energy source, so eat up!

***Complex carbohydrates* - grains and starch**

Beans, brown rice, couscous, long grain rice, quinoa, wild rice

Corn, potatoes, sweet potatoes, yams

Oatmeal, whole grain bread, pasta, wraps

Fats

Fish: High-fat varieties listed above

Avocado, olives, nuts, nut butter with no added sugar, seeds (sunflower, chia, flax)

Cold-pressed oils: avocado, olive, sesame

MY WELL-STOCKED KITCHEN

I try to have the following things on hand or on my grocery list to re-stock:

Pantry:

- Canned beans, chickpeas
- Canned tomatoes
- Beef, chicken, veggie broth
- Dry beans
- Oatmeal
- Rice
- Quinoa
- Vinegar
- Olive & avocado oil
- Olives

- Pickles
- Canned Tuna- packed in water

Refrigerator:

- Eggs
- Cheese
- Salsa
- Lemons

Freezer

- Whole grain bread & tortillas
- Fruit
- Vegetables

BALANCED EXAMPLES

Breakfast Options:

1. Scrambled eggs with fruit or oatmeal or toast
2. Scrambled eggs with veggies
3. Protein smoothie with fruit and nut butter
4. Cottage cheese with fruit
5. Greek yogurt with fruit and pecans
6. Egg sandwich

Snack Options:

1. Turkey, fruit, and nuts
2. Edamame
3. Turkey, fruit, and cheese
4. Greek yogurt dip and apple + veggies
5. Cottage cheese with fruit + veggies

Lunch/Dinner Options:

1. Chicken salad
2. Turkey burger with veggies
3. Tuna salad with fruit + veggies

4. Chicken fajita
5. Sushi
6. Salmon with brown rice, asparagus
7. Grilled chicken with raw spinach, garbanzo beans, balsamic dressing
8. Steak with sweet potato and steamed cauliflower
9. Scallops with cooked brown rice and green beans
10. Shrimp with broccoli and quinoa
11. Sirloin steak with veggie salad and roasted cauliflower
12. Grilled burger with a whole wheat sandwich thin, lettuce, tomato, and onion

Late Snack:

1. Cottage cheese and raw veggies
2. "Nice" cream

COOK ONCE- EAT AGAIN

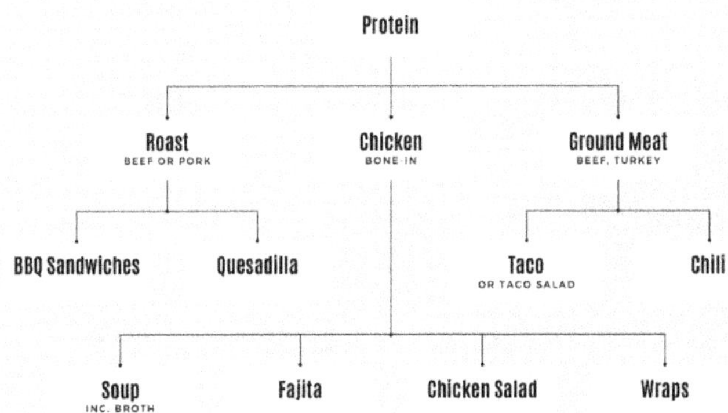

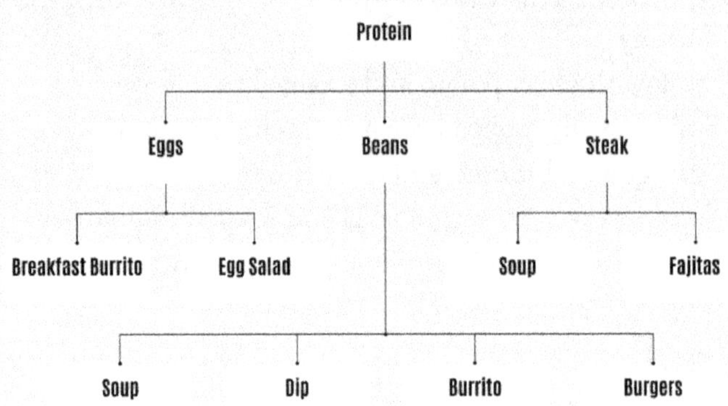
COOK ONCE- EAT AGAIN & AGAIN!
Protein
Eggs
Beans
Steak
Breakfast Burrito
Egg Salad
Soup
Fajitas
Soup
Dip
Burrito
Burgers

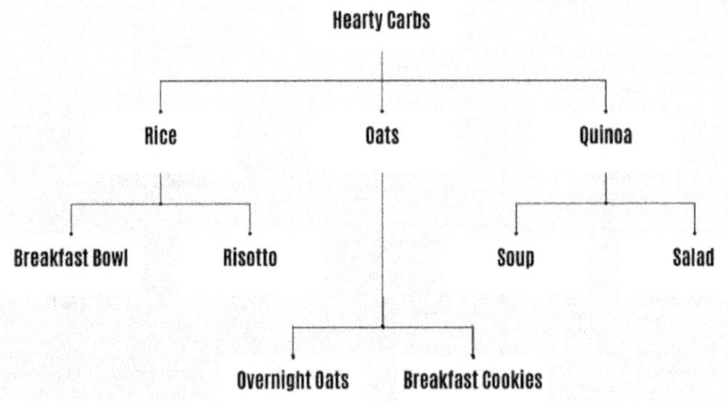
COOK ONCE- EAT AGAIN & AGAIN!
Hearty Carbs
Rice
Oats
Quinoa
Breakfast Bowl
Risotto
Soup
Salad
Overnight Oats
Breakfast Cookies

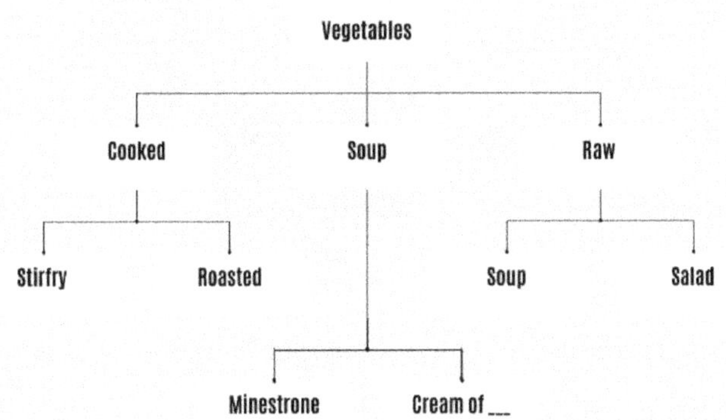

PLANNED LEFTOVERS

Mexican Pot Roast Tacos

3-pound beef shoulder or chuck roast

1 tsp black pepper

2 cloves garlic, minced

1 onion, sliced

28 oz can crushed tomatoes

1 Tbs chile powder

1 tsp cayenne pepper

1 Tbs ground cumin

3 bay leaves

1. Place all ingredients in a slow cooker (or a gallon-sized bag to freeze for another day).
2. Refrigerate or freeze (if freezing, thaw in fridge for at least 24 hours before cooking)

Cooking Day:

1. Place in slow cooker on Low for 7-8 hours
2. Remove meat and bay leaves.
3. Shred the meat and put it back in the sauce- toss bay leaves in the trash.
4. Prepare using tortillas with your favorite toppings

Option: serve over rice or make oven nachos

Thai Steak

This is a single recipe- I like to double it for fajitas later in the week!

1 ½ lb. flank or sirloin steak- 1" thick

Juice of half a fresh lemon

¼ cup olive oil

¼ cup fresh chopped cilantro or parsley

2 cloves garlic, minced

Dash of hot sauce

3 tsp honey or agave nectar

½ tsp sea salt

½ tsp black pepper

1. Place steak in a large baking dish.
2. Mix all other ingredients in a mason jar. Tighten the lid. Shake well.
3. Pour over the steak. Cover and let marinate for several hours.
4. Grill on high heat- first side 2 minutes.
5. Turn the grill to indirect heat for 7-9 minutes longer to the desired doneness.
6. Let rest for 5 minutes.
7. Slice thinly across the grain.

Marinated Chicken 2 Ways!

Mustard Marinated Chicken:

¼ cup cider vinegar

3 Tbs whole-grain mustard

3 cloves garlic, peeled and minced

1 lime, juiced

½ lemon, juiced

¼ cup brown sugar

½ tsp salt

5 Tbs olive oil

Ground black pepper

6 boneless skinless chicken breast halves

1. Whisk ingredients (cider vinegar through salt) in a large glass container.
2. Whisk in olive oil and pepper.
3. Place chicken in the mixture.
4. Cover and marinate chicken in the fridge for 8 hours or overnight.
5. Remove chicken from the marinade just before you turn on your grill or broiler to let it come up a few degrees. **Discard marinade.**
6. Lightly oil your grill or broiler pan.
7. Grill or broil about 7-8 minutes per side.

Chipotle Lime Chicken

½ cup olive oil

Juice of 2 limes

1 tsp chipotle powder

2 cloves garlic, peeled and minced

½ tsp sea salt

ground pepper to taste

6 boneless chicken breast halves

1. In a large, non-reactive container, whisk together ingredients through pepper.
2. Place chicken in the mixture.
3. Cover and marinate chicken in the fridge for 8 hours or overnight.
4. Remove chicken from the marinade just before you turn on your grill or broiler to let it come up a few degrees. **Discard marinade.**
5. Lightly oil your grill or broiler pan.
6. Grill or broil about 7-8 minutes per side.

Pork Carnitas

3-4 pounds boneless pork loin roast

ground black pepper

2 tsp dried oregano

1 tsp ground cumin

2 Tbs olive oil

1 onion, coarsely chopped

4 cloves garlic, minced

1 jalapeno, seeded and ribs removed, chopped

1 orange, cut in half

½ cup water

1. Pat the roast with dry paper towels.
2. Season with pepper
3. Mix the oregano and the cumin with olive oil and rub all over the pork.
4. Place the pork in a slow cooker and top with the onion, garlic, and jalapeno.
5. Squeeze over the juice of the orange and add the two halves.
6. Add water.

7. Cover and cook on low for 7- 8 hours.
8. Once the meat is tender, remove it from the slow cooker and let it cool slightly before pulling it apart with a fork.

Beans in Instant Pot

1 pound of dried beans rinsed and sorted

Boiling water to cover

—

8 cups water

1 bay leaf, optional

1 onion, diced, optional

2 cloves garlic, peeled and whole

1. Place rinsed beans into an Instant pot, with boiling water to cover the beans.
   Close the lid and let it rest for 45 minutes.
2. Drain beans and return them to the IP with water, garlic, onion, and a bay leaf.
3. Place the lid on the Instant Pot and close the valve to "seal."
4. Cook on High Pressure for the following times:

- Black, navy, or kidney beans--25 Minutes on High Pressure
- Chickpeas--30 Minutes on High Pressure

*Add 10 minutes if you want them softer for dip or soup.

5. Allow to release naturally until pressure subsides, or at least 20 minutes before doing a quick release.
6. Store cooked beans in a glass jar covered with the cooking liquid.

SOME OF MY FAVORITE RECIPES

SEASONINGS

Fajita seasoning

3 tsp chili powder

2 tsp paprika

1 tsp onion powder

1 tsp. garlic powder

1 tsp cumin

½ tsp cayenne

Place spices in a small jar with a lid and shake until mixed.

Taco Seasoning

¼ cup chili powder

¼ cup cumin powder

1 Tbs garlic powder

1 Tbs onion powder

1 tsp ground oregano

1 tsp paprika

1 tsp sea salt (optional)

1 tsp ground pepper

Place spices in a small jar with a lid and shake until mixed.

Sprinkle on ground beef or chicken like any store-bought taco seasoning.

3 tablespoons is the same as 1 packet of store-bought taco seasoning.

BREAKFAST

Banana Muffin Pancakes

½ cup old-fashioned oats

½ banana, mashed

¼ cup cottage cheese

1 egg

½ tsp cinnamon

Blend ingredients and cook on a hot griddle. Flip when set and bubbling in the middle

*Recipe is 2 servings

Breakfast Burrito

1 lb breakfast sausage

2 Tbs oil- if needed

1 onion, diced

1 bell pepper, diced

½ tsp salt

½ tsp pepper

12 large eggs

8 large flour tortillas (burrito size)

½ cup shredded cheddar

1. Crumble sausage and cook until no pink remains. Remove sausage to a medium bowl.
2. Wipe excess grease from the pan. If the sausage is very lean, heat oil.
3. Add the onion and bell pepper to the pan. Season with salt and pepper.
4. Sauté over medium heat until the onions are soft and translucent (about 5 minutes).
5. Add the bell pepper and onion to the sausage. Set aside.

6. Crack 12 eggs into a bowl and lightly whisk. Pour into the hot skillet.
7. Stir eggs until most of them have set, but the eggs still look moist. Do not overcook!
8. Add eggs to the sausage mixture. Stir to combine.
9. Add a scoop of sausage/ egg mixture to the middle of each tortilla, then sprinkle with a tablespoon of cheddar cheese.
10. To roll the burritos, fold the tortilla up from the bottom, then fold it in the sides, and then finish rolling it up until it has closed. Wrap each burrito in parchment paper.
11. Lay flat and slightly spaced on a baking sheet and place in the freezer for 3 hours
12. Transfer the frozen burritos to freezer bags, label, and date the bags, then store them in the freezer.

Two ways to reheat!

1. Transfer the breakfast burrito to the refrigerator the night before to thaw. Microwave on high for 1-2 minutes, or heat in a skillet over medium-low, about 5 minutes on each side, or until the insides are warm.
2. To reheat from frozen, defrost in the microwave for 3 minutes, then microwave on high for 1-2 minutes or until heated through.

Egg and Spinach Quiche Cups

10 ounces frozen chopped spinach

1 dozen eggs

½ cup shredded cheese

2 large mushrooms diced

½ cup red bell pepper, chopped

½ cup onion, chopped fine

Hot sauce (optional)

1. Microwave the spinach on high for 2 1⁄2 minutes. Drain well and press with whitepaper towels until most of the liquid is removed.
2. Line a 12-cup muffin tray with foil baking cups. Spray the cups with cooking spray.
3. Whisk eggs in a large bowl.
4. Combine the eggs, cheese, mushrooms, peppers, spinach, and onions in a bowl.
5. Add hot sauce (or salt and pepper) to taste.
6. Divide evenly among the cups.
7. Bake at 350 for 20 minutes or until a knife inserted comes out clean.
8. Enjoy, or refrigerate/freeze in a large freezer bag for another day.

To reheat: Reheat in the microwave for 30 seconds.

To heat from frozen, microwave for 1-2 minutes.

Company Worthy Oatmeal

3 cups old-fashioned oats

3 cups vanilla almond milk

3 cups water

2 Tbs pure vanilla extract

1. Spray slow cooker with non-stick spray.
2. Combine all ingredients and stir to mix.
3. Cover and cook on low for 4-6 hours. (Perfect to start right before bed!)
4. Before serving: Stir. If it is too thick, add some hot water. If too thin, turn to HIGH for 30 minutes, stirring occasionally.
5. Serve in bowls and top with roasted berries and protein yogurt (recipe below)

Roasted Summer Berries

7 cups mixed berries (I used what I had on hand: 1 pint blackberries, 1 pint red raspberries,

1 pint blueberries, 4 cups THAWED frozen mixed berries)

1. Rinse the berries if fresh and put them in a large-rimmed baking sheet or shallow casserole.

2. Roast in a preheated 400° oven for 30 minutes.

The berries will break down and make a thick syrup.

Protein Spiked Greek Yogurt

1 ½ cups Greek or Icelandic Vanilla yogurt

3 Tbs vanilla protein powder.

1 Tbs almond milk (if needed)

1. Combine ingredients in a small bowl and whip until combined.

To serve- layer 1⁄2 cup oatmeal, 1⁄4 cup berries, and 1⁄4 cup yogurt mixture. Enjoy!

SNACKS & APPETIZERS

No-Bake Protein Bars

2 cups old-fashioned oats

½ cup natural peanut butter

4 scoops protein powder (chocolate or vanilla)

1 Tbs ground flaxseed

½ cup water

1. Knead all ingredients in a large bowl
2. Line 8x8 baking pan with wax paper. Spread dough into the pan.
3. Freeze for 30 minutes.
4. Remove from the freezer and cut into bars. Makes 16.

Salsa Dip

½ cup cottage cheese

½ cup salsa

½ cup plain fat-free yogurt

1 jalapeno, seeded and chopped

1. Blend and refrigerate. Mix before using.

Ranch Dip

1 cup cottage cheese

1 green onion, chopped

Ranch seasoning to taste

Ground black pepper to taste

1. Combine the cottage cheese and green onion and blend for about 30 seconds.
2. Add the ranch seasoning and pepper to taste.

PB-Greek Yogurt Dip

1 cup plain Fat-Free Greek yogurt

$^{1}/_{3}$ cup natural creamy peanut butter

1. Mix well. Serve with apple slices or celery.

Lite Avocado Dip

1 ½ cups of green peas, fresh or frozen, cooked and cooled

1 avocado, seeded and chopped

1 clove of garlic

1 Tbs lime juice

hot sauce to taste

1. Place all the ingredients into a food processor and mix to your preferred consistency.

Crispy Garlic Parmesan Edamame

1 package frozen shelled edamame, thawed

1 Tbs olive oil

¼ cup grated parmesan cheese

¼ tsp garlic powder

salt and pepper to taste

1. Preheat the oven to 400 degrees.
2. Dry the edamame on a paper towel if necessary.
3. Mix parmesan cheese, garlic powder, salt, and pepper in a bowl.
4. In a separate bowl, toss edamame with olive oil.
5. Add the parmesan-spice mixture to the edamame and toss until evenly coated.
6. Spread onto the pan and bake for 15 minutes (until the cheese is crispy).

Taco Dip This is one of my favorite party recipes!

8 oz. Philadelphia cream cheese

8 oz. plain Greek yogurt

16 oz. jar mild salsa

3 Tbs taco seasoning recipe (from above) or 1 packet

2 cups romaine lettuce, shredded

2 large tomatoes, diced

1 cup shredded cheddar cheese

½ cup sliced black olives

½ cup sliced green onions

1. In a large bowl, combine cream cheese, sour cream, salsa, and taco seasoning and mix well with an electric mixer.
2. Spread on the bottom of a large shallow glass dish.
3. Top with shredded lettuce, tomatoes, shredded cheese, onions, and black olives.
4. Serve with baked tortilla chips.

Healthy Hummus

1- 15-ounce can chickpeas, rinsed and drained well

Juice from 1 lemon

¾ teaspoon salt

2 cloves garlic, very finely minced

¼ cup plain yogurt

3 Tbs extra virgin olive oil

½ tsp smoked paprika

Combine chickpeas, lemon juice, salt, garlic, and yogurt in a food processor.

Process for 1 minute, then open the food processor and scrape the sides, process for another minute.

While the processor is running, pour in the olive oil.

Taste and check for a smooth consistency. If the hummus is too thick, add 1 tablespoon of water.

Just before serving, sprinkle with smoked paprika

Spiced Nuts and Seeds

3 cups whole nuts (almonds, pecans, walnuts, pistachios)

1 cup roasted soy nuts

¼ cup each flaxseed

¼ cup sunflower seeds

¼ cup pumpkin seeds

2 egg whites

2 Tbs honey or maple syrup

1 ½ tsp coarse salt

¼ tsp cayenne

¼ tsp cumin

¼ tsp cinnamon

1. In a large bowl, combine nuts and seeds
2. Whisk egg whites with honey, salt, cayenne, cumin, and cinnamon in a separate bowl.
3. Toss with nut mix.
4. Spread in a single layer on a baking sheet; bake at 325° until dry, stirring occasionally, about 30 minutes.
5. Scrape from pan while cooling to avoid sticking. Makes 16 servings

SOUPS

The Best Soup Ever

Shared with me many years ago, and it is still one of my favorites! Thanks, Sherri!

2 lbs ground turkey or lean beef

1 onion, diced

3 carrots, chopped

3 stalks celery, chopped

3 cloves garlic, minced

2- 14.5 oz can of diced tomatoes

1 15 oz can of red kidney beans

1 15 oz great northern beans

1 15 oz can of no-sugar tomato sauce + 1 can of water

1 Tbs Balsamic vinegar

1 tsp oregano

1 tsp basil

1 tsp thyme

Salt and pepper to taste

1. Brown the meat, drain it, and set it aside.
2. In a large soup pot, saute the onions, carrots, celery, and garlic in olive oil until the onions soften.
3. Add the meat to the pot.
4. Add the remaining ingredients and simmer for at least 30 minutes.
5. You can modify this recipe in many ways: add bell peppers, mixed frozen vegetables, or zucchini.

* you can also combine ingredients in a slow cooker after step 1. Cook on low for 4-6 hours.

As with many soups, it tastes even better the next day!

Italian Wedding Soup

2 lbs lean ground meat (I like a mix of turkey and mild Italian sausage)

2 eggs, slightly beaten

¼ cup dry oatmeal

1 Tbs parmesan cheese

1 tsp dried Italian seasoning

½ tsp onion powder

2 Tbs olive oil

2 carrots, finely chopped

1 small onion, finely chopped

2 stalks celery, finely chopped

1 Tbs dried Italian seasoning

8 cups low-sodium chicken broth

2 cups chopped escarole or spinach

½ cup orzo pasta, uncooked

1. Bring a large pot of water to a boil.
2. In a medium bowl, combine meat, egg, bread crumbs, parmesan cheese, Italian seasoning & onion powder; shape into ½" balls. (Use a melon ball tool or similar utensil to ensure consistent size).
3. Drop meatballs, one at a time, into boiling water. Allow room for them to float freely, cooking in several batches. Remove from boiling water with a slotted spoon to a cooling rack. Allow water to return to a boil before cooking more meatballs.
4. In a large saucepan, heat olive oil. Saute carrots, onions and celery until tender. Add broth and heat to boiling; stir in spinach and orzo. Drop cooked meatballs in a few at a time.
5. Return to boil; reduce heat to medium.
6. Cook at a slow boil for 10 minutes or until the orzo is tender. You may have to add more broth to thin the soup to the

desired consistency. (I like to use the meatball cooking liquid) Stir frequently to avoid sticking.

Slow Cooker Chicken Taco Soup

1 onion, chopped

1-16oz. can of chili beans or pinto beans (don't rinse)

1- 15oz. can black beans (don't rinse)

1- 15oz. can whole kernel corn, drained

1- 8 oz. can tomato sauce

2- 10oz. cans of diced tomatoes with green chilies, undrained

3 Tbs taco seasoning (recipe above), or one packet

1 tsp garlic powder

1 tsp chili powder

1 tsp cumin

2 cups chicken broth

3 whole skinless, boneless chicken breasts

1. Place the onion, chili beans, black beans, corn, tomato sauce, chicken broth, and diced tomatoes in a slow cooker.
2. Add all seasonings. Mix well.
3. Lay chicken breasts on top of the mixture, pressing down slightly until just covered by broth.
4. Set the slow cooker on low heat, cover it, and cook it for 5-7 hours.
5. After cooking, the chicken should be tender enough to shred with two forks.
6. Mix into soup. Keep warm until served.

Slow Cooker Chicken, Mushroom and Wild Rice Soup

1 medium onion, chopped

3 carrots, peeled and chopped

3 stalks celery, chopped

2 cloves garlic, finely chopped

8 oz. thinly sliced Shiitake mushrooms

1 cup uncooked wild rice, rinsed and drained

2 bay leaves

½ teaspoon dried thyme

Salt and pepper, to taste

2 Tbs Mrs. Dash Grilled Chicken Seasoning

3 skinless chicken breasts and 3 skinless chicken thighs (2-2 1⁄2 pounds)

10 cups low-sodium chicken broth, divided

½ cup plain Greek yogurt or sour cream

1. In a 6-quart slow cooker, combine onion, carrots, celery, garlic, mushrooms, wild rice, bay leaves, thyme, salt, and pepper. Top with chicken. Add 8 cups of chicken broth.
2. Place the lid on the slow cooker and cook on low heat for 6 to 6 1/2 hours.
3. Carefully remove the chicken and shred it with two forks. Return to the slow cooker and stir. Remove the bay leaves.
4. Whisk the remaining 2 cups of chicken broth into 1⁄2 cup plain Greek yogurt in a separate bowl. Stir the yogurt mixture into the soup.

MAIN DISHES

I don't follow a lot of recipes. I've fallen into a rhythm of putting things together as I go because of how I stock my kitchen. The following are three recipes we love and enjoy frequently!

Turkey Roll-Ups

This is my go-to recipe when I want to take a meal to someone. I adapted the original recipe from *Clean Eating Magazine*[1] to be a little more "saucy" and spicy. Imagine a delicious lasagna perfectly portioned into a single serving size. Snuggle as many as you can in your baking dish- I can fit 12 rolls into a 9x13 pan. I almost always make an extra casserole for dinner or to freeze for another day.

1 Tbs olive oil

1 small chopped onion

1 clove minced garlic

2 lb Italian turkey sausage, ground or removed from casings (I like a mix of sweet and hot)

¾ tsp ground cinnamon

1/4 tsp ground nutmeg

1 -28-oz can whole tomatoes

1 jar of no-sugar spaghetti sauce

16 sheets whole wheat lasagna noodles

2 boxes frozen chopped spinach, thawed and drained

1 ½ -15oz. containers of low-fat ricotta cheese

2 eggs

2 cups shredded reduced-fat mozzarella

1. In a large skillet, heat oil. Add onion and cook until softened, about 5 minutes. Add garlic and cook for another minute. Add ground turkey sausage- cook until meat shows no sign of pink. Stir in cinnamon and nutmeg, then add tomatoes (crush when you add) and pasta sauce. Reduce heat to medium-low, stir, cover, and let simmer for 20 minutes, stirring occasionally.

2. Meanwhile, bring a large pot of water to boil. Cook pasta according to directions. Remove sheets to a bowl of ice water when al dente, then spread out on large, clean flour sack towels.
3. Squeeze all remaining moisture from thawed spinach and place in a large bowl. Add ricotta, egg, and 1 cup of mozzarella. Stir until combined.
4. Spread 2 cups of cooked tomato sauce onto the bottom of a casserole dish. Lay a cooked noodle flat in front of you. Use your fingers to spread ¼ cup of ricotta mixture across the noodle and roll it up. Place rolled pasta, seam side down, into the casserole dish. Repeat with remaining noodles. Spread remaining sauce over roll-ups, then top with remaining ½ cup mozzarella.
5. Bake, covered with foil, for 20 minutes. Remove foil and broil for 5 minutes or until roll-ups are browned and bubbly.

Stuffed Peppers

1 lb. ground beef, cooked

1 cup brown rice, cooked

4 large bell peppers

1 cup Parmesan cheese

1 ½ cups no-sugar spaghetti sauce

2 garlic cloves, minced

1 tsp salt

1 tsp pepper

1 cup shredded Mozzarella cheese

1. In a large pot, brown ground beef. Rinse and drain.
2. Remove and discard the tops and seeds of the peppers and level the bottom so they sit flat.
3. Mix beef, rice, parmesan, 1 cup of spaghetti sauce, garlic, salt, and pepper in a bowl.
4. Spoon an equal amount of the mixture into each hollowed pepper.

5. Place stuffed peppers in a square baking dish standing upright .

This can be frozen at this point! Cover with foil and freeze.

1. If baking right away, pour ¼ cup spaghetti sauce over the stuffed peppers.
2. Bake covered at 350 degrees for 1 hour or until peppers are tender.
3. Remove cover, sprinkle peppers with cheese, and bake for five more minutes uncovered or until cheese is melted.

IF FROZEN:

1. Thaw overnight.
2. Remove foil, pour ¼ cup spaghetti sauce over peppers, and cook as above.

Crustless Pizza

1 package pepperoni

1 lb Italian sausage, crumbled and cooked

3 cups mozzarella cheese, divided

3 cups veggie, diced- we used a mix of bell peppers, onions, olives, mushrooms

1 ½ cups tomato sauce

1. Preheat oven to 400°.
2. Line the bottom and sides of a 9 x 13 casserole dish with pepperoni.
3. Sprinkle 1 ½ cups cheese over pepperoni.
4. Layer in order: sausage, tomato sauce, veggies, remaining cheese.
5. Cover with foil and bake for 20 minutes.
6. Remove foil and bake for an additional 20 minutes.
7. Let sit for 5-10 minutes, slice and enjoy.

BEVERAGES

Shrubs - My new go-to favorite mocktails are created with homemade shrubs. Shrubs are drinking vinegars, and I love them because they're so easy to make and showcase the very best fruits in season.

I've included three of my favorites, but you could use almost any fresh or frozen fruit (except melons), spice, or flavoring to create a drink that's perfect for you! The directions are the same for all the shrubs- let me know if you make a flavor you love!

Blueberry Ginger Shrub

1 cup granulated monk fruit sweetener (regular cane sugar can be used as well)

1 cup water

2 cups fresh or frozen blueberries

½» x 3» slice of ginger, sliced

Rind from 2 lemons

1 cup apple cider vinegar

LemonThyme Shrub

1 cup granulated monk fruit sweetener (regular cane sugar can be used as well)

1 cup water

3 lemons, scrubbed and sliced into rounds

3 sprigs of fresh thyme

1 cup apple cider vinegar

Black Cherry Pepper Shrub

1 cup granulated monk fruit sweetener (regular cane sugar can be used as well)

1 cup water

2 cups black cherries, pitted

1 TBS. black peppercorns

½ vanilla bean

1 cup apple cider vinegar

Directions for making shrubs:

1. Heat the monk fruit sweetener in water until it is completely dissolved.
2. Add the fruit and spices.
3. Simmer for 15 minutes.
4. Pour all ingredients into a large glass canning jar and let cool.
5. Add the apple cider vinegar and cover with a lid.
6. Refrigerate for 24-48 hours.
7. Strain fruit and store the shrub in the fridge for (up to) 6 months.

To serve, pour 2 oz shrub over ice, top with tonic, soda, or flavored sparkling water, and squeeze your favorite citrus! Shrub is also delicious in lemonade or iced tea or drizzled over ice cream ☺

DESSERTS

Cran-Pine-Apple Crisp for a crowd

5 large Granny Smith apples- peeled, cored, and cut into 1/2" size chunks

1 medium, ripe pineapple- cleaned, cored, and cubed into 1" pieces- JUICE RESERVED!!

1 ½ cups whole cranberries

2 cups old-fashioned oats

¼ cup coconut sugar (raw sugar or brown sugar work as well)

1 cup flaked coconut

3 Tbs melted butter or coconut oil

Reserved pineapple juice- add water or apple cider to equal 1/3 cup

½ cup chopped pecans (optional)

1. Preheat the oven to 350°.
2. Spray a large 9×13 casserole dish with non-stick spray.
3. Mix prepped fruit in the dish.
4. Mix oats, sugar, coconut, and pecans (if using) in a bowl.
5. Drizzle melted butter and juice on the oat mixture and mix well with your hands.
6. Spread oats evenly on the fruit.
7. Bake in a preheated oven for 40-50 minutes.
8. Serve warm with vanilla Greek yogurt, whipped cream, or ice cream.

Pumpkin Custard

I stumbled upon this recipe from the book *Prairie Home Cooking* by Judith Fertig[2] when making my first "from scratch" pumpkin pie one Thanksgiving. I had more filling than the crust would hold, and I decided to bake it in ramekins for a post-holiday treat. It has become my go-to pumpkin recipe- I think it's better without the crust!

3 cups pumpkin, freshly cooked or canned puree

4 eggs, lightly beaten

1 cup half & half

¾ cups honey

1 tsp cinnamon

½ tsp nutmeg

½ tsp salt

1. Mix all ingredients in a large mixing bowl.
2. Pour into a lightly sprayed 2-quart casserole dish.
3. Place the casserole in a larger baking dish and fill the outside dish with hot water to the custard line.
4. Bake at 325° for 75-90 minutes or until a knife comes out of the center clean.

You can also bake in individual-sized ramekins. The recipe will make about 10.

Cook in a water bath, but reduce cooking time to 45 minutes.

Top with vanilla Greek yogurt, vanilla ice cream, or whipped cream.

Any Fruit Frozen Yogurt

I love to use fruit at the peak of its flavor. My favorites this summer have been cantaloupe and peach. If you use fruit at its best, you'll rarely need additional sweetener.

4 cups frozen fruit

½ cup plain Greek yogurt

Optional: vanilla extract, honey, peanut butter, and yogurt flavors.

1. In the bowl of a food processor, combine the frozen fruit and Greek yogurt.
2. Process the mixture until it is creamy, about 5 minutes.

Serve immediately or transfer it to an airtight container and freeze it until ready to serve.

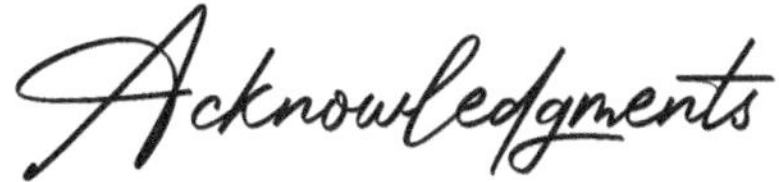

Embarking on the journey of writing this book has been a profound experience.

There have been numerous unexpected twists and challenges since I first dared to pull words from my journals. Looking back, I am genuinely appreciative of each detour and roadblock.

The book before me today surpasses the one that initially took shape in my mind many months ago.

Many thanks…

Jeff, my unwavering pillar of support... your belief in me and support in bringing my dreams to life are true gifts. My deepest love, forever and ever.

Zachary and Samuel, you are my greatest blessings, and I thank God for you every day. You remain my most cherished creations, and I will love you always.

Kat and Madi, thank you for continuing where I left off, loving my boys the way I prayed someone would, and for being the daughters I always dreamed of... I love you.

Brooks, Baby C, and all the future littles in my life, I will always love you to the moon and back (plus just a little more). Thank you for the opportunity to embark on yet another journey.

My parents, all four of you, I love each one of you more than you know. Thank you for your wisdom, patience, and unconditional love.

Mardi and Sandy, you took a chance all those years ago. The example you set every day in your gym made me a better coach, and I am forever grateful.

Alison, Amy, Deb, Heather & Jon, Jennifer, Katie, Kaylen, Lisa, Sherri, Susan, and Taylor, and countless others whose examples and stories may not grace the pages of this book: I am deeply thankful for your trust, friendship, and inspiration.

Amy, Christy, Jenna, Kim, Krissi, and Roberta: thank you for your experience and willingness to share your expertise with me. The work you do every day empowers women to live their best lives. Thank you!

Christine, Jessica, Jody, Lea, Lisa, Karen, and Rachel: your early suggestions, even when the words were still finding their way, were instrumental in shaping something I will forever be proud of. Thank you!

Alane, your coaching pulled me out of a creative rut! Your wisdom and faith helped me find clarity in my jumbled thoughts. Thank you.

I thank Brian for your vision, Krissy for your leadership, Tj for sifting through the rough patches and bad words, Kati for polishing the good words, Hope for your patience and amazing organizational skills, and the whole team at Hope*Books for bringing my dream to reality.

To the incredible men and women in my Hope*Books cohort: You have been the best part of this experience! I am in awe of your stories and vulnerability as we waded through this process together. I can't wait to meet you in "real life" and to add your books to my collection.

Danny, Haley, Carrie, Pete, Nicole, and Sarah: Thank you for the way you love Jesus and for providing the opportunities I needed to re-open the door to His Love.

And finally, to the One who has always loved me, I offer my thanks. I pray the words you placed on my heart resonate with women everywhere.

Citations

Introduction

1. Good News Network, "'Don't Be Afraid of Your Fears. They're Not There to Scare You. They're There to Let You Know That Something Is Worth It.' – C. JoyBell C.," *Good News Network*, November 21, 2020, https://www.goodnewsnetwork.org/c-joybell-c-quote-about-fear/.
2. Integrative Nutrition, "Why Crowding Out Is the Healthiest Way to Diet," Institute for Integrative Nutrition, March 4, 2021, https://www.integrativenutrition.com/blog/2016/10/why-crowding-out-is-the-healthiest-way-to-diet.

Chapter 1

1. Thomas Fleet, *New England Primer* (1750), 23.
2. Richard J. Foster, *Prayer: Finding the Heart's True Home*, (New York: HarperOne, 2009), 349.
3. Becky Tirabassi, *Let Prayer Change Your Life* (Becky Tirabassi, 2011).
4. Staci Salazar and Staci Salazar, "Don't Underestimate the Value of Doing Nothing," Our Family Lifestyle, March 3, 2020, https://ourfamilylifestyle.com/value-of-doing-nothing/.
5. Jennifer Tucker, *Breath as Prayer* (Nashville, Tennessee: Thomas Nelson, 2022).
6. Danáe Ashley, "Spiritual Direction vs. Therapy: What Is the Difference?," Faith+Lead, September 10, 2022, https://faithlead.org/blog/spiritual-direction-vs-therapy-what-is-the-difference/.
7. Jennifer Tucker, *Breath As Prayer* (Nashville, Tennessee: Thomas Nelson, 2022), 32.
8. Cultivate, "Write the Word Journals," n.d., https://cultivatewhatmatters.com/collections/write-the-word.

Chapter 2

1. Reddit.com//r/quotes (8/23/15)
2. Julia Cameron, *The Artist's Way* (New York: TarcherPerigee, 2016), 3. Reddit.com//r/quotes (8/23/15)
3. Ibid.
4. "NaNoWriMo," n.d., https://nanowrimo.org/.

Chapter 3

1. Scott Erickson, *Happy Advent* (Grand Rapids, Michigan: Zondervan, 2020), 98–99.
2. "Image Consultants and Personal Stylist Specialists in the USA | House Of Colour," n.d., https://www.houseofcolour.com/.
3. Ibid.
4. "Image Consultants and Personal Stylist Specialists in the USA | House Of Colour," n.d., https://www.houseofcolour.com/.
5. Ibid.

Chapter 4

1. "Jules Robson Quotes," Jules Robson Quotes, accessed November 5, 2023, https://i-love-motivational-quotes.org/author/jules-robson.
2. "Exercise: How Much Do I Need Every Day?" Mayo Clinic, July 26, 2023, https://www.mayoclinic.org/healthy-lifestyle/fitness/expert-answers/exercise/faq-20057916.
3. Ibid.
4. "Exercise and Physical Activity," National Institute on Aging, n.d., https://www.nia.nih.gov/health/topics/exercise-and-physical-activity.

Chapter 5

1. "Default - Stanford Medicine Children's Health," n.d., https://www.stanfordchildrens.org/en/topic/default?id=the-benefits-of-mothers-own-milk-90-P02339.
2. Evelyn Tribole and Elyse Resch, *Intuitive Eating* (New York: St. Martin's Essentials, 2020).

3. National Eating Disorders Association, "National Eating Disorders Association," n.d., http://www.nationaleatingdisorders.org/.
4. "Standard American Diet," NutritionFacts.org, n.d., https://nutritionfacts.org/topics/standard-american-diet.
5. Janet L. Yellen, "The History of Women's Work and Wages and How It Has Created Success for Us All | Brookings," Brookings, January 6, 2021, https://www.brookings.edu/essay/the-history-of-womens-work-and-wages-and-how-it-has-created-success-for-us-all/.
6. Centers for Disease Control and Prevention, "ADHD throughout the Years," CDC, September 27, 2023, https://www.cdc.gov/ncbddd/adhd/timeline.html.
7. ADDitude Editors, "ADHD Statistics: New ADD Facts and Research," ADDitude, June 28, 2023, https://www.additudemag.com/statistics-of-adhd/.
8. Ibid.
9. Autism Community In Action, "Autism Prevalence Is Now 1 in 44, Signifying the Eighth Increase in Prevalence Rates Reported by the CDC Since 2000," *Cision PR Newswire*, December 2, 2021, https://www.prnewswire.com/news-releases/autism-prevalence-is-now-1-in-44-signifying-the-eighth-increase-in-prevalence-rates-reported-by-the-cdc-since-2000-301436766.html.
10. "National and State Diabetes Trends | CDC," n.d., https://www.cdc.gov/diabetes/library/reports/reportcard/national-state-diabetes-trends.html.
11. USAFacts, "US Obesity Rates Have Tripled over the Last 60 Years," USAFacts, April 26, 2023, https://usafacts.org/articles/obesity-rate-nearly-triples-united-states-over-last-50-years/.
12. Kira Sampson and Gazettebeckycoleman, "Dramatic Rise in Cancer in People under 50," *Harvard Gazette*, November 9, 2023, https://news.harvard.edu/gazette/story/2022/09/researchers-report-dramatic-rise-in-early-onset-cancers/.

13. World Health Organization: WHO, "Infertility," April 3, 2023, https://www.who.int/news-room/fact-sheets/detail/infertility.
14. Dan Buettner, *The Blue Zones American Kitchen* (Washington, DC: National Geographic, 2022), 22.
15. "Nutrition and Weight Management | Boston Medical Center," Boston Medical Center, n.d., https://www.bmc.org/nutrition-and-weight-management#:~:text=An%20estimated%2045%20million%20Americans,Americans%20are%20overweight%20or%20obese.

Chapter 6

1. Nikol Chen, "Every Great Dream Begins with a Dreamer," Laidlaw Scholars Network, August 6, 2021, https://laidlawscholars.network/posts/every-great-dream-begins-with-a-dreamer.
2. "Spaghetti Saturdays," Veggies by Candlelight, n.d., https://www.veggiesbycandlelight.com/spaghetti-saturdays-post/.
3. https://www.neighborstable.com/
4. "Iron Chef America," Food Network, n.d., https://www.foodnetwork.com/shows/iron-chef-america.
5. "The Family Freezer," The Family Freezer, n.d., https://thefamilyfreezer.com/.

Chapter 7

1. "Raise the Bar Initiative," Raise the Bar Initiative, n.d., https://www.raisethebarinitiative.com/.
2. Stacy Westfall, ""Sometimes You Find Yourself in the Middle of Nowhere and Sometimes in the Middle of Nowhere You Find Yourself." - Official Site of Stacy Westfall," Official Site of Stacy Westfall, August 2, 2017, https://stacywestfall.com/sometimes-you-find-yourself-in-the-middle-of-nowhere-and-sometimes-in-the-middle-of-nowhere-you-find-yourself/.
3. "More Giving Quotes to Inspire and Remind Us That Giving Matters! - 365give," 365give, July 27, 2018, https://365give.ca/more-giving-quotes-to-inspire-and-remind-us-that-

giving-matters/.https://www.bluezones.com/2017/01/blue-zone-2017/.

4. Aislinn Kotifani, "5 Easy Steps to Blue Zone Your 2017," Blue Zones (blog), July 27, 2023, https://www.bluezones.com/2017/01/blue-zone-2017/.
5. Craig M. Hales, Jennifer Servais, Crescent B. Martin, and Dafna Kohen, "Prescription Drug Use among Adults Aged 40–79 in the United States and Canada," CDC, August 14, 2019, https://www.cdc.gov/nchs/products/databriefs/db347.htm.
6. Ibid.
7. "SoberSIS - Sober Minded Sisterhood," n.d., https://www.sobersis.com/ss-home.
8. "Have a Problem with Alcohol? There Is a Solution. | Alcoholics Anonymous," n.d., https://www.aa.org/.
9. "Home - Celebrate Recovery®," n.d., https://www.celebraterecovery.com/.
10. "How to Drink Less or Quit Drinking Alcohol," n.d., https://www.ditchedthedrink.com/.
11. "SAMHSA - Substance Abuse and Mental Health Services Administration," SAMHSA - the Substance Abuse Mental Health Services Administration, n.d., https://www.samhsa.gov/.

Conclusion

1. Andy Frisella, *75 Hard* (Andy Frisella, 2020).

Back of the Book

1. "Hydrant | Hydration Packets for Water," Hydrant, n.d., https://www.drinkhydrant.com/.
2. "Your Daily Superblend," Ka'Chava, n.d., https://www.kachava.com/.
3. "TÖST - Sparkling Alcohol-Free Beverages," TÖST, n.d., https://tostbeverages.com/.
4. Curious Elixirs, "CURIOUS ELIXIRS | Booze-Free Craft Cocktails | Non-Alcoholic Beverages – Curious Elixirs," n.d., https://curiouselixirs.com/.

5. Clean Eating Magazine, https://www.cleaneatingmag.com/recipes/pasta-roll-ups-with-turkey-and-spinach/

6. Judith M. Fertig, *Prairie Home Cooking* (Beverly, Massachusetts: The Harvard Common Press, 1999), 389.

www.ingramcontent.com/pod-product-compliance
Lightning Source LLC
Chambersburg PA
CBHW022049020426
42335CB00012B/605
* 9 7 9 8 8 9 1 8 5 0 3 0 9 *